MW01230097

YOU'RE PREGNANT, NOW WHAT?

A Simple Guide to a Healthy Pregnancy and Faster Recovery

Kaitlin E. Spano PPCES, M.Ed

ISBN 979-8-89043-533-0 (paperback)
ISBN 979-8-89043-534-7 (digital)

Christian Faith Publishing
832 Park Avenue
Meadville, PA 16335
www.christianfaithpublishing.com

Printed in the United States of America

For Christie, my best friend, who lost her life bringing her baby into the world.

Contents

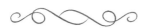

Foreword

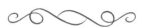

"You're going to do great! It's going to be OK and you'll be holding your baby boy soon, I love you and I can't wait to see pictures."

As I hung up the phone late that Friday evening, I was feeling excited, impatient and also irritated that I lived about 5 hours away from my best friend. Christie was not just my best friend, she was my soul sister and the connection we had was what I had always dreamed of having in a sister after having only brothers growing up (five of them nonetheless).

She was in labor with her first baby, a boy, and unfortunately she had been laboring over 20 hours (or more, I can't exactly remember). She was on pitocin and things didn't seem to be progressing as she had hoped. A cesarean was not her ideal birth but the doctors were telling her it was probably best at this point.

She called me before they prepped her for surgery, as we were states apart, and she was scared. I told her it was going to be OK, that it was all going to be OK.

Throughout that night I thought of her, waiting for my phone to ring or ping with a picture of her & her baby boy. By mid morning that following day my phone was ringing from an unknown number, I immediately knew it was Christie calling me from the hospital to share the exciting news.

I answered, "Christie!"

On the other line "Hello, Kaitlin? Is this Kaitlin?"

"Yes, this is her."

"Oh, Kaitlin, Hi, this is Maureen, Christie's mom…"

"Oh yes, Hi! How is she?! How are you?!…"

"Well….ummm…Christie didn't make it."

Audible *GASP*

"Umm, wait, WHAT? Um, wh… what?!"

"Oh, Kaitlin, she had the c-section but she didn't make it. Her baby is OK, but she didn't make it…and, and I knew I had to call you right away because she loved you so much & I wanted to tell you…" …silence.

I could hear the thump, thump of my heart beating louder and louder into my ears as it quickly turned into a ringing sound, my breath quicked…what do I say? What in the hell do I say?! My mind instantly became a murky, cloudy mess.

…this clearly all had to be a dream and not happening I told myself. The feeling of doom instantly radiated through my stomach as it drove bile up to my mouth. I was going to vomit.

I'm not exactly sure what happened after that moment, I said some things to her mom but I truly don't remember what I said after hearing those four words…" she didn't make it." I remember calling my husband at work, calling my mom, then falling onto the floor gasping for air to fill my lungs, not really understanding the degree of what just transpired.

This all cannot be true I told myself, the last thing I told her was that she was going to be OK.

This is not OK…

She is not OK…

She is not OK!!!

If I was there could I have stopped this?

What could have stopped this?!

This single moment changed the trajectory of my future pregnancies, how I viewed pregnancy, pregnant people and the birth experience.

As I became pregnant with my first only 4 months after Christie passed, I began to research pregnancy, birth and recovery from a place of fear. I was fearful, I was scared, how do I have a successful pregnancy and not die? How can I prevent a c-section, why do they happen? What if I die too? How can I prepare my body so I can be ready for this big event?

Through this continued research over the last decade I have learned that our bodies are so intricately designed to give life and as a society we don't honor that enough. Our bodies were so beautifully designed to stretch, grow, and birth our babies, yet there is a large gray area around the pregnant body and how it works. For some unambiguous reason, this information is not shared with us.

Don't we deserve more than this?

We have been giving birth since the beginning of time, so why is this information about our bodies not mainstreamed or shared to every woman who becomes pregnant?

I truly believe that if my best friend had access to this information her outcome could have been different & she would still be here today, yet if she was still here…would I have done this research and written this book for you?

With the knowledge you are about to learn, it is my hope that you will feel confident, empowered and strong as you navigate the beautiful changes that unfold through the season of pregnancy and motherhood.

Knowledge is power, and this power can help you make decisions and choices about your body and birth with confidence as you embark upon this journey.

To more empowered, confident pregnancies and births,
XO
Kaitlin

Introduction

When you first become pregnant, you become overrun with a multitude of emotions. Maybe this has been a challenging journey for you (if it has been, please know that I am here, holding you in my thoughts), maybe this was unexpected, or maybe it was planned and is turning out exactly as you intended. Regardless of how it happened, it has happened, and this is such a special time in your life. You want to do everything you can to have a healthy pregnancy, keeping yourself and your baby as healthy as possible.

Unfortunately, as a society, we are so overrun with either too much information that is not accurate or not enough information at all. Women are still being told to just do Kegels to prepare for their pregnancy, that back pain can't be helped during pregnancy, that leaking is normal after a baby, and some things are just a right to motherhood.

You (we) deserve more than this.

You're Pregnant, Now What? A Simple Guide to a Healthy Pregnancy and Faster Recovery is based on research and facts that your doctor is more than likely not providing for you. Now, I am not saying that *all* doctors withhold this information from their patients, but it is also safe to say, it is not exactly under the umbrella of your doctor to inform you of all the information you are about to learn. Their main concern is to check for abnormalities, difficulties, high-risk pregnancies, and make sure your pregnancy is progressing with no abnormalities within the medical umbrella.

With that being said, the United States also has the *highest* rate of maternal deaths *per capita* despite being the country that spends the most on its health care. Seeing as my best friend now sits in this statistic, you bet your bottom, I'm going to work as hard as I can to change that.

Unfortunately, birth has become very robotic, and as a society, we have come too far away from the simple act of positive noninvasive births. Many factors have come into play to get to this robotic point. The first step to change is knowledge and understanding of how your body works and how to keep it healthy during the special season of pregnancy and postpartum through research and evidence-based care.

It is hard to find research and evidence-based care related to pregnancy and postpartum when looking because most of it is left in lengthy reports that are hard to decipher; and frankly reading long lengthy reports when you become pregnant is probably the very last thing on your mind.

What is evidence-based care? you may ask. Evidence-based care is the combination of best research evidence with clinical experience and the patients values and preferences. In other terms, it means receiving accurate, evidence-based information to help you make decisions by a professional who is paying attention to these practices and cares about your values and preferences as an individual.

The problem with this is that it takes fifteen to twenty years to get that evidence and education into practice. There are many fantastic providers out there who are doing their best to put evidence-based information out there, while others have been slower to make the switch. There are several reasons for this. Some don't know that it is available to them. They don't believe it. They don't think it will change anything, or they don't want to go against the status quo.

Which is why, I'm here to break this all down for you because you, my friend, are worthy of understanding exactly what the evidence-based information is and how your body works during pregnancy and after. God designed our bodies so incredibly amazing. (I mean, think about it; our babies will grow fingers, toes, hair, ears, and more without us having to put much thought into it.)

You deserve to know how to keep your body functioning and feeling your best during this very special season of pregnancy and postpartum. Pregnancy and postpartum are a *season* and need to be treated as such. There are varying degrees of what needs to be done, when, and *this* is what our society lacks greatly on telling us. This book is here to be your guide in all these loopholes!

After birthing five babies in a short span of six years (my oldest had not turned six yet when I had baby number five!), I realized how much my movement journey during pregnancy and the "body after baby" evolved over time and how *not* to look at it. Society has taken prey on mothers after they have babies (and it honestly starts *during pregnancy*), and I was one of them.

Let's change this course. We are not and should not be victims of our body image, nor should we be stuck in a body that does not function because "that is what happens when you have a baby," or the "eventually, you will start to feel better" system. The information coming out on how to fill that postpartum gap starts right here with preparing your body for a healthy pregnancy, labor, and birth. It starts with filling the pregnancy gap and helping mothers understand exactly how to navigate the changes that take place during pregnancy.

This book will show you exactly what you need to focus on to prepare your body for pregnancy, labor, birth, and recovery so you can be successful with your pregnancy journey and beyond baby. With that being said, there is a lot of information here. Don't let it overwhelm or stress you; it just means, there is room for change and growth.

Who is this book for?

This book is for anyone who is preparing for a baby, is pregnant with a baby, or has had a baby. Whether you are preparing and reading this pregnant, just had a baby, or are years or decades out from having a baby, this book is for you. This book is also for anyone who works or supports (fitness trainers, yoga/Pilates instructors, midwives, doulas, nurses, mental health clinicians, social workers, physical therapists, etc.) pregnant or postpartum women.

The information present is going to allow you to see your body from the inside out to understand its intricate detail that was so beautifully designed to create babies. When you tap into what God gave you, you will be amazed at what you can accomplish.

Part 1

Requirements for Movement during Pregnancy and Why It Matters

When we are trying to conceive or become pregnant, we all have high hopes and big dreams for it to be the best experience ever. We want to stay fit, feel confident, and radiate with that pregnancy glow. Then reality sets in; you are exhausted beyond belief, the all-day nausea, the smell of certain foods completely turns your stomach, you have constant headaches and body aches, and you are feeling less than stellar. This is not what you imagined, and the thought of performing any sort of extracurricular routine feels daunting and out of the question.

In general, the Centers of Disease Control and Prevention (CDC) recommends 150 minutes of moderate-to-intense aerobic activity and two days of strength-based movement each week for a non-natal person. Aerobic means activity that supports your heart such as walking, jogging, or biking. Strength-based movement means to build and keep muscle mass, such as Pilates, barre, or any strength-bearing moves. Why is this important? Because our bodies need daily movement to stay healthy, stay strong, keep up with our kids, and so we can live our daily lives to the best of our abilities.

During pregnancy, there is a small shift in requirements because the demands on our body change. Our body physically changes—from our heart to our muscles to our internal organs. Your heart literally changes shape, becoming larger to accommodate the increase of blood flow and oxygen in your body. How miraculous is this?!

The American Center of Obstetrics and Gynecology also recommends 150 minutes per week of moderate aerobic activity and at least two days of strength-based movement for the pregnant individual. The difference here is the word *intense* is removed from the requirements during pregnancy. As you read this, 150 minutes per week may feel like a lot, but if you break it down, it can look like 30 minutes of walking for five days (which can further be broken down into 10-minute sessions) and two days of 20-minute strength sessions. That seems much more manageable, doesn't it?

As a pregnant mother (and after the baby comes), you need to build and maintain strength so you can carry the weight of your baby, keep your stability, and prepare for the demands of motherhood and your everyday life. I like to refer to this as functional movement. We have to learn to move effectively in our everyday life to prepare our bodies for birth (y'all, birth is a major life event) and for the constant demands of motherhood. We have to hold our babies for endless hours, rock them, coddle them, pick up their car seat, carry all the bags, carry the groceries, do the laundry, carry our toddlers, put them in the bath, and the list will go on and on and on.

Overall, movement (aerobic and strength training) is important for longevity and longtime health as a person. Staying active during pregnancy supports not only your well-being but also the health of your baby. The issue with staying active during pregnancy is that our doctors don't give us much to go by or how to make it work for us. We are given these recommendations that feel overwhelming and not possible for us to achieve, so we head to the Internet and find that most of the programs out there are intimidating, out of reach, and not designed for the changes of the pregnant body. We become overwhelmed and stuck on how to move forward, so we generally toss the whole notion out the window, thinking, "I am not that person. I can't do this." (I promise you can, and the rest of this book will show you how!)

However, we do know that taking part in these weekly movement activities can:

- reduce back pain;
- ease constipation;
- reduce pregnancy-related conditions such as pre-eclampsia, gestational diabetes, and the need for a cesarean section;
- promote healthy weight gain during pregnancy;
- increase overall mood;
- support postpartum mood disorders; and
- increase the overall health of your baby from brain to heart.

As long as you have the clear from your doctor to exercise, any bit you can do will be positive for you and your baby.

Functional movement during pregnancy should be low-impact and leave you feeling energized, strong, and ready for your day. Workouts should not deplete you or leave you in pain. Through this book, I share exactly how to do simple, beginner-level moves in your daily life that will prepare you for a healthy pregnancy, labor, birth, and motherhood journey. These moves will leave you feeling energized, strong, stable, and best of all, you will feel confident knowing that the moves you are doing are based on the simple science of a changing mother's body during pregnancy and postpartum.

So let's get to it, shall we?

Part 2

Pregnancy

Eighty-five percent of women will carry a child at some point in their life, which means many of us have already gone through the changes, are going through them, or plan to go through them. The changes that take place during this forty-week span is miraculous. (Truly, God knew exactly what he was doing, making a pregnancy last this long.) There is no other way to put it. The fact that we, women, can become pregnant and then the baby grows all needed body parts while we just motor along, envisioning what this little human will look like is a *big deal*.

As much as we would like to control certain things about our growing baby inside of us, we can't. There are many things during pregnancy that are out of our control in which we have to let faith or fate or whatever you believe to roll out in this process.

However, what we *can* control is how we approach our pregnancy. That comes with understanding the exact changes that our bodies will go through at this time, how to keep ourselves feeling our very best, and how to prepare our bodies for our best birth and birth recovery. So let's get this party started, yea? There is a reason pregnancy is, on average, forty weeks long; that is because this allows us ample time to prepare our mind and body to birth a baby and to recover. Some of you reading this might assume that preparing for a healthy pregnancy means running four miles a day or spending hours in the gym, or lifting weights. However, not everyone wants to lift weights, and that is okay. If you refer back a few pages where I shared what the recommendations were for strength-based movement, it was a minimum of twice a week. You can build and keep muscle with bodyweight movement only. This is a great place to start, and you need minimal equipment—only your body! Using your body weight will support that functional fitness needed for motherhood that I mentioned previously while checking those boxes to keep you strong and healthy for this season of life.

For many of us, we feel that we want to do everything possible to prepare our bodies and keep our little one safe growing inside of us, but we have no idea where to start. Maybe you are a fitness guru and want to run as long as you can during pregnancy, or maybe you have had a hard time keeping a consistent routine in the past, and the thought of starting one now seems silly and overwhelming. Again, let's throw that notion out the window. When you understand your body, what changes during pregnancy, and how to build strength within these specific areas, then preparing for a healthy pregnancy becomes simple and achievable.

Cesarean birth rates are on the rise with the United States having the highest rate in the world. In 2011, one in three women had a cesarean birth. It has become noted that there is an overuse of cesareans as the data is showing an increase in variation and not a clear reason as to why a cesarean birth was performed. Some of the reasons a cesarean birth is given is due to lack of dilation, labor not progressing, change in a baby's heart rate, a breech baby, and various other emergencies. Part of the increase in cesarean birth rates are a failure on the overall health care system and the lack of information that is provided for our pregnant mothers. Some of this has come from the overuse of mechanized birthing tactics, lack of supportive care, and the health care system as a whole.

Women are *not* provided with information on how to work *with* their bodies during labor. For instance, I have heard stories of women asking questions about birthing their baby on all fours to their obstetrician. The response of the OB was that they must be on their back because any other way could be fatal. This is fear-based doctoring, and it is not necessary. Women should be encouraged to learn about their bodies and how to use other birthing positions to support the delivery of their baby.

Whether a pregnant mother chooses a home birth or a hospital birth, both should encourage and support a woman's body mechanics and use this to encourage labor and delivery with the least interventions possible. I do think there is a lot of positive work happening to support women during labor and birth, but so much work still needs to be done. What is that wise old saying? "Nothing changes if nothing changes."

Now let me state that cesareans *are* important. Thirty-three percent of women give birth by cesarean. There is absolutely nothing wrong with this. For many mothers and babies, this is what needed to happen to have a safe birth. There are very critical periods of timing that must be performed to save baby and mom; I am not here shaming them. I think women who birth via cesarean are extremely strong; and their recovery is unlike anything else.

However, the data is showing that the system is turning to this form of delivery over vaginal birth with no clear reasoning. If you look at the trends of cesarean births throughout the year, you will see that they rise right before a national holiday or right after. Interesting fact, isn't it? We know that a baby comes when the baby wants; however, with this data trend, it is clear that women are being induced right before or right after holidays, increasing the rate of unneeded cesareans at this time.

The biggest issue with the increase with cesarean births is that it is a major abdominal surgery, and it increases the risk of complications. Mothers who have a cesarean are not being supported for their recovery, and this leads to trauma and complications further on in a woman's life. There is a framework that I am going to share with you that will support your body holistically to prepare your body and mind for birth so you can be empowered in your choices.

The four-part framework to prepare your body for pregnancy, birth, and beyond:

1. Functional body mechanics
2. Nutrition
3. Mindfulness
4. Birth prep

We are going to break down each of these sections so you can take away simple action steps to prepare your body for a healthy pregnancy, labor, birth, and beyond.

Pregnancy presents a biomechanical change in your body, period. Whether you are a seasoned athlete or have never picked up a dumbbell before in your life, your body *will* experience these changes. No one is immune to these changes; they all happen because our bodies were so wonderfully designed to create life.

Let's first review functional body mechanics as this is the largest chunk to understand. There are six foundations within this pillar that are the building blocks to understand and prepare your body for pregnancy. Once you have an understanding of these six foundations, you can apply them to your daily life during pregnancy and beyond.

Core four

Your core four is made up of four primary muscles that surround the center of your body, the exact place where we grow a small human.

The core four muscles are made up of your diaphragm (image 1), your transverse abdominis, your pelvic floor, and a small but mighty muscle that runs along your spine called your multifidus. All four of these muscles must work in unison to have a properly working core unit. Why do you need a properly working core unit? Well, because your core four is your center and dictates all your other movements you do daily.

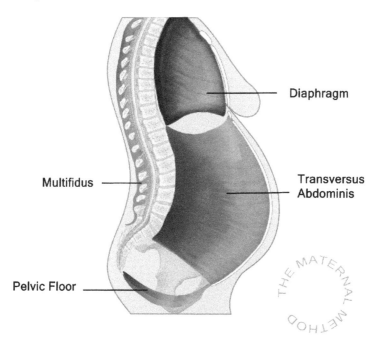

Diaphragm

Multifidus

Transversus Abdominis

Pelvic Floor

Think of a car. If your pistons do not go up and down correctly, your entire car will not run properly. Your body works the same way. If you are not activating your breath correctly, which activates your entire core four system, the rest of your body cannot function and do what it is meant to do.

Now the reality of it is, ninety-five percent of our population is *not* using their core four muscles correctly. Layer a pregnancy over that, and you've got a whole system that needs some fine-tuning.

So back to the top, your diaphragm is where we need to breathe from. You take on average twenty-five thousand breaths a day. Your transverse abdominis is your innermost core muscle. It connects from your diaphragm, wrapping all the way around to your spine, down to your pelvic floor. Your transverse is literally a corset that keeps you stable in your everyday life. Your uterus lies just under your transverse. Imagine, as your pregnancy progresses, the amount of stretch and lengthening that muscle does throughout your pregnancy. You have four layers of muscles within your core (image 2).

On top of your transverse lies your inner obliques, which run diagonally, your external obliques, and at the very top of your core unit, you have your rectus abdominus. The rectus abdominis muscles are the ones that many can see on a human if they have a very low body fat percentage and are otherwise known as a six-pack. Now all these muscles are encased with a nice layer of what we call fascia. We will learn more about this later in this book, but I wanted to mention it because you can see it clearly in the visual provided for you here.

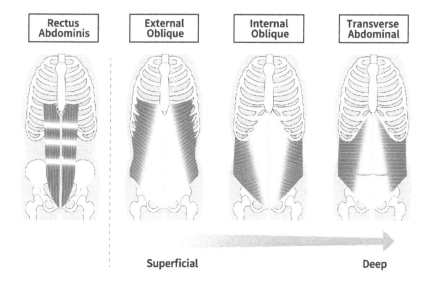

Let's review:

- Your core four is made of a dynamic system of muscles that all need to work together.
- Your core four is the powerhouse of your body and needs to be strengthened specifically.
- Pregnancy puts stress on your core four and will cause it dysfunction.

Diaphragmatic breathing

Believe it or not, our diaphragm is the muscle that allows us to take our twenty-five thousand breaths each day; our lungs are what filter the air. The diaphragm is the main muscle in taking a full expansive inhale and exhale. Despite the fact that we take on average twenty-five thousand breaths each day, literally, without much thought, the majority of us lose our natural breath patterns over time.

11

Pregnancy happens to be one of those times, which is why it is critical to understand how to bring your body back to its natural state of breathing. Ninety-five percent of us, when we become pregnant, are out of our natural alignment and breathing patterns, which puts us at a disadvantage as our bodies change course over the pregnancy. When we are babies, toddlers, and children, our bodies breathe and function the way it was intended. As we become adults, stress begins to enter into our lives, we have an injury or become pregnant, and these natural breathing patterns become out of sync. We start turning into chest breathers, also known as shallow breathers. When we breathe through our chest, taking shallow breaths, it signals to our brain that we are stressed and puts our body into a fight-or-flight mode.

There is actually research that states that the left side of our nostril is responsible for fight-or-flight feelings in the body and activates more of the right side of the brain, while the right side is more responsible for stress relief and the left side of the brain. (*Breath*, Nestor)

Not only is breathing a wild and wonderful coping mechanism/healing tool that has been long lost and forgotten about, it is also the one tool that will support you the most in your pregnancy, labor, and birth journey.

The importance of breathing through your diaphragm is that each piece of your core four is properly engaged, allowing the pressure inside of your abdomen to be equalized through each breath. This means that all your surrounding muscles are also doing what they need to do, which will minimize low-back pain, neck pain, or even shoulder pain you may experience during pregnancy. Correct breathing through your diaphragm also signals to our brain the "I feel good. I don't feel stressed. I'm getting more oxygen to my blood, which means more oxygen to my brain, therefore I feel less stress."

If you have an infant or toddler in your home, I really encourage you to watch them breathe and see how their ribcage/stomach moves when they take a breath. More than likely, you will see that their rib cage expands open, and then their abdomen expands down and out, and then it contracts in and up on the exhale. This is what we call a diaphragmatic breath!

Understanding how to breathe through your diaphragm relating to pregnancy is essential because you're going to have times where you feel very stressed, especially when you experience labor. (We will discuss this more in the birth prep section.) When we breathe the way that our body was designed to, believe it or not, it automatically begins to eliminate pain in our bodies because our bodies are now functioning the way that they were meant to function.

Let me give you an example, one that I actually give to my husband many times throughout the week. Say you are home from a long day at work and are feeling tension and tightness in your neck/shoulder area, or maybe it is your lower back (a very common pain point for pregnant women). I challenge you to take five minutes to focus on your breathing and breath into the part of your body that is causing you tension. Do this for five minutes or so, and let me know how you feel! With that being said, I am going to walk you through exactly how to take a diaphragmatic breath to begin feeling all these amazing, feel-good feelings (image 3).

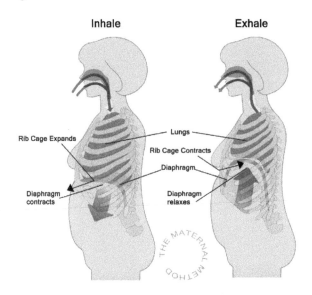

Inhale   Exhale

How to breathe through your diaphragm:

Step 1: Let's start by putting your hands on your lower rib cage, right under your breasts. If it is comfortable, you could lie down or sit cross-legged on your bed. As you inhale (through your nose), expand through the sides and back of your rib cage, you should feel your rib cage pushing against your hands at this point.

Step 2: As you are inhaling, you will feel your lower belly expand (don't force anything) allow the air to go down through your abdomen and down to your pelvic floor.

Step 3: On the exhale (out your mouth), your rib cage will now close inward. You should feel them pull away from your hands. As this happens, your pelvic floor will slowly come up. (This is not a Kegel or a contraction!) Your abdomen will tighten, and the very top of your rib cage should come in and close. Phew! That, my friends, is a diaphragmatic breath.

Now do that five to ten times, and tell me you don't feel calm, cool, and relaxed. This is how God designed our bodies to work. But that does not mean it is going to be easy, especially if your body has not been optimizing proper breathing patterns. Keep coming back to this time and time again, and soon enough you can reestablish proper breathing patterns. A great time to practice this is before you get out of bed in the morning, at some point in the middle of the day, and before you go to bed again.

Note: It's really important to understand that a diaphragmatic breath is not any sort of contraction or muscle flex. You are not doing a Kegel with your pelvic floor; you're not contracting your abdomen; it truly is just a flow of your breath in and out. We will discuss more of an actual contraction of your pelvic floor with your diaphragm and your transverse abdominis when we discuss how to perform a belly pump later in this book. Onto the next amazing piece of our body: your pelvic floor!

Let's review:

- Breathing through your diaphragm helps regulate normal bodily functions.
- It has a direct effect on the pressure, pushing out on your abdominal wall, low back, and pelvic floor.
- Breathing through your diaphragm is the first step to reducing pregnancy ailments and aiding your body during labor.
- Practice this method for ten breaths before you get out of bed, during the middle of your day, and before you go to sleep.

Pelvic floor

We all have a pelvic floor, male and female alike. During pregnancy, your pelvic floor has to bear the weight of your growing baby, and it stretches fifty times its size to accommodate the birth of your baby. Now that is a miracle.

So what exactly is your pelvic floor? Your pelvic floor is a group of muscles, not one singular but a group of eight muscles that sit at the base of your core four unit (image 4). Your pelvic floor supports your lower organs, keeping them up and in, such as your anus and vagina. Your pelvic floor helps to control urination, bowl movements, sexual function, and it helps keep you stabilized in your daily movements.

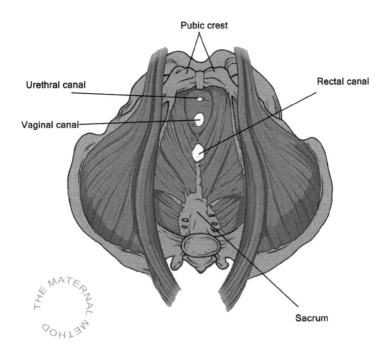

These eight muscles that make up your pelvic floor are intertwined with several other muscles, which make it the powerhouse or center of your daily bodily movements. In the front of your pubic bone, your pelvic floor muscles are connected up to your transverse abdominis. In that pelvic region, the muscles connect to each of your sitz bones on the side and then connect up to your sacrum, which you most likely know as your tailbone.

Your pelvic floor is also connected to your glute muscles and your inner thigh and outer thigh muscles. It is so interconnected to so many muscles, which is why, just doing Kegels is an extremely inaccurate information to pregnant or postnatal woman, or any women in general! Doing Kegels in isolation does have a time and place, but when performing them in isolation, you are leaving out all the other stabilizing muscles mentioned above. Doing only isolated Kegels during pregnancy or postpartum will increase imbalances, causing aches and pains.

Now that you have a much better understanding of how your pelvic floor is connected to all these vital points, you can see how important your pelvic floor is for stabilization in your daily movements.

Understanding beyond the Kegel is important because we need to understand that our pelvic floor naturally moves with each breath we take. With this understanding, we can then learn how to strengthen and lengthen our pelvic floor like any other muscle in our body.

The strengthening plays a part in keeping your body strong and stabilized while your center of gravity changes during the pregnancy period. During pregnancy, as your center of gravity changes, your pelvic floor, hips, and low back will "lock" up, for lack of a better term, because your body is trying to keep everything stable and upright. This lockup causes your muscles to be in constant tension, which brings about the common aches and pains of pregnancy. This is where correct strengthening of the pelvic floor and the interconnected transverse abdominus, glutes, inner thighs, and hip strengthening play a vital role in reducing the common aches and pains associated with pregnancy.

The lengthening part is extremely important because our baby will pass through our pelvic floor during birth (unless it is a cesarean birth, but your pelvic floor is *still* affected regardless of how you birth). Remember what I said before that the pelvic floor will stretch fifty times its size during childbirth.

It is critical to understand how to open and lengthen our pelvic muscles so our baby can come down through the birth canal. Doing Kegels in isolation causes a tight pelvic floor, which will make it hard to relax as the baby descends down. We will review more of this as I guide you through birth preparation practices later in this book.

Let's review:

- Your pelvic floor is the base of your core four unit. It is a group of muscles that acts as a hammock to your inner organs.
- As pregnancy progresses, the weight of your baby pushes on this, which could cause heaviness, leaking, and pressure.
- Proper strengthening and lengthening of this muscle is very important during pregnancy, and it is more involved than a single Kegel isolation.

Transversus abdominis

Your transversus abdominis, or what I will refer to as TVA throughout the rest of this book, plays an integral part in your pregnancy and postpartum movement journey as you have started to see how interconnected all these muscles are in our core unit (image 5).

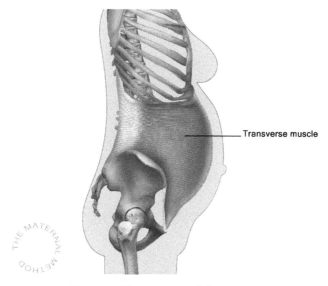

(Image 5: Transversus Abdominis)

I always tell my clients that postpartum healing begins during pregnancy. If you want to have a faster recovery, understand this information now so you know the exact steps to healing after the baby.

Your TVA is your innermost abdominal muscle (see image 5), and it is the one that is attached to your upper rib cage. It goes down around your back and attaches to your spine along your tailbone and connects right in front to your pelvic floor. It truly is a very, very large center muscle that provides you much of your stability.

Your TVA muscle supports your body's breathing process through the diaphragm by supporting the exhalation part of your breath. It also provides some minor compression to your intestinal tract, which is really needed to support healthy digestion and help with bowl movements. Being aware of this during pregnancy will support you that much more in your postpartum journey.

Why is your TVA important?

Your TVA is important because it is the muscle that supports your entire core unit. It works in unison with your pelvic floor and your diaphragm, which I mentioned before. It stabilizes your back, pelvis, and it must fire before you perform any movement as it is the base of your stability structure. The main function of your TVA is to activate the core muscles as a whole and stabilize your pelvis and lower back prior to any movement or loading in your body.

Regardless of what you're doing, whether you are exercising or running (either to exercise or after your children!), whether you're picking up a car seat, picking up a toddler, reaching for a book on the floor, reaching above your head for something on the shelves, twisting to reach a kid in the back seat of your car, or any of those things, your TVA and entire core four unit need to be functioning and firing on all these moves. Again, when we were babies, toddlers, and young children, these muscles would do what was intended. It is over time, as we sit more, look at our phones, walk less, move less, or become pregnant, our stabilizing unit becomes weakened and needs reminders how to work together.

When your TVA is activated correctly, it efficiently allows the rest of your body to stay in a neutral position as you put any type of load onto it. Your TVA supports your correct posture alignment, which is essential especially as a prenatal or postnatal individual. Your TVA supports your balance, stability, and ladies, it is the main muscle to support in guiding your baby out during birth with contractions.

Another reason your TVA is vitally important to activate and strengthen during pregnancy is that it helps you control your intra-abdominal pressure throughout pregnancy, which can support in the reduction of a diastasis once you have the baby. (More on this in the postnatal section.)

When you understand how to properly engage your entire core four, your body can go back to moving and stabilizing the way it was intended. So many times, what happens is, we are not even aware of these muscles or that we should be activating a certain way to keep them a well-oiled machine. I mean, when I first learned this information, my mind was exploding (insert that little mind-blown emoji).

During pregnancy, especially during the second and third trimesters, there is so much internal pressure and pushing taking place from the growing baby. This pressure inside of our core four system will either push up, down, or out if we are not making it a point to equalize said pressure.

This is where the aches and pains begin and where complications can arise post baby. The pressure could push too much on your pelvic floor, which may cause the leaking or the low back pain. The pressure could be going out incorrectly through your midline fascia, which could be the result of a hernia, injury-based diastasis, or excess stretching in general.

So how do I make sure I am doing this correctly, Kaitlin? How? Correct activation of your TVA is done through—you'll be shocked, I know—*correct breathing through your diaphragm!* This is where I am going to warn you to be wary of what you see people out there on social media and the fitness industry telling you. Nothing irritates me more when large-scale fitness leaders (even those who claim to be prenatal/postnatal certified) cue you to suck in your core, pull your belly button to spine, or demonstrate on video a completely inaccurate representation of TVA breathing. I am very passionate about this subject and am certified in very specific perinatal processes for this specific reason.

I just want to interject quickly here that when I was expecting my second son, I had debilitating back pain in my right side. I mean, walking up my driveway, chasing my one-year-old would bring me to tears. As a former marathon runner, this was obviously a very, very humbling moment for me. My OB continued to tell me it was part of being pregnant. I went to the chiropractor. They took pictures of me, told me my posture was awful, that I was leaning one way and would be a good candidate to get some help.

So twice a week I would go down there. They would put me on their inversion table thingy, use a special gun in a matter of minutes, and send me on my way. Not once did they explain to me how my posture should look, how I should stand. The only thing they told me (I was teaching preschool part-time at the time, plus I had my one-year-old) was to not sit on the floor. I mean, *y'all*, looking back now, I am embarrassed for them and sad for me and all the other women who may have had encounters similar to this. How was any of this truly helpful? How our bodies function throughout our day is what affects us the most and what is important to be aware of.

With that being said, I am going to accurately tell you how to engage your TVA within your core four unit. And if you begin to feel any slight back pain coming on while pregnant, go back to these basic foundations and *breathe*.

Proper core activation with the TVA subconsciously will take place before any lifting movement, or as one physical therapist in this industry stated, it's the "blow before you go." When you first practice this, which is referred to as the belly pump (fit for birth), you can be lying down or sitting crisscross on the floor or on a chair, whatever is most comfortable for you. This belly pump is what I like to refer to as your active core breathing. You are engaging all muscles in your core four to support proper activation in your core unit and to strengthen all noted muscles. The belly pump, or active core breath is what you will perform during daily movement exercises or at those times of picking up your kiddo, lifting your laundry basket, or anytime you are putting a load on your body.

How to perform a belly pump:

1. As you inhale through your nose, release your abdomen and pelvic floor while expanding your rib cage laterally. Think of filling a balloon with air.

2. On the exhale, you will tighten up from the bottom of your core unit so you are lifting your pelvic floor in and up, wrapping your deep core from your pubic bone (think hip bones closing and zipping up through your belly button, wrapping all the way up to tighten and close your rib cage).

3. Connecting and strengthening your transverse abdominis in this way takes practice. It is a mind-muscle connection that we have become out of touch with in our daily movements. The longer you have been unaware of this connection, the longer it's going to take for you to recalibrate that mind-muscle connection. The more you practice, the stronger your core will become, the stronger you will become in all movement areas of your pregnancy and postpartum season, which will take you through the rest of your life!

Strengthening your TVA is the backbone of preparing and staying strong for your pregnancy and postpartum recovery. This is information that is based on best practice and the science of functional movement. When you have a strong core unit, understanding how to connect to it is going to reduce pain in your pregnancy journey and allow you to recover faster postbaby.

Let's review:

- TVA is the muscle that supports your entire core unit as it wraps around your entire center.
- The main function of your TVA is to activate the core muscles as a whole, to stabilize the low back and pelvis prior to any other movement.
- The belly pump is the exercise that supports the strengthening of your TVA and allows you to control your inner pressure.

Alignment/posture

The other piece to reducing pain during pregnancy and postpartum and keeping your core unit functioning correctly is having proper alignment (image 6).

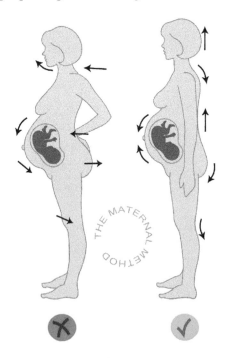

Engaging your TVA and having the correct core activation is only one piece of the puzzle. Shockingly enough, your posture is going to improve the more that you begin this corrective exercise of strengthening your deep core and breathing through your diaphragm. Being aware and conscious of how your body is positioned and understanding how to keep yourself stacked with a neutral pelvis is one way to reduce aches and pain for you during your pregnancy and postpartum experience.

Posture matters during pregnancy because as your body grows and adapts to accommodate and make room for the baby, your center of gravity is changing. Maintaining proper strength, posture, and alignment is going to provide the least amount of pain and pressure on your joints and especially your low back. Most of us experience low back pain because our core is not firing correctly, so our backs have overcompensated for our weak core.

The main thing that I want you to take away from this on alignment and posture is understanding neutral. Having a neutral pelvis is so important for you to understand. When your pelvis is in a neutral position, which I'll explain a little bit more, you are in alignment. Your body can function correctly the way that it was made. In today's society, we have become so far away from how a neutral alignment looks and feels like due to screen time. When we are on computers, our necks are protruding forward, and our shoulders are slumping along for the ride. We are sitting more, so it automatically puts our pelvis at this weird anterior tilt. Especially for moms carrying kids, we tend to put them on one side of our body and our hips push out one way. We stand leaning one way or the other or have to lean on objects. This could be due to the fact that our core unit is weak. I am not saying you specifically have a weak core, but this is what comes up time and time again in this practice. This affects our everyday functioning and aches and pains we may be feeling all throughout our bodies.

How to understand neutral pelvis

I want you to think of neutral like this: Think that your pelvis/hip area is a bowl, and it's full of some water. So you're holding that bowl in front of your hips. During pregnancy, we tend to get the anterior tilt so our butt pops out backward; your belly pops forward. As that happens, your bowl of water is going to tip and splash out the front.

This is what we don't want! After we have a baby, we tend to be stuck in that anterior tilt, or we push back into a posterior tilt (image 6). This is when we push our bum too far forward to balance the baby on our hips or the laundry basket or all the bags we now have to carry. This is going to make the bowl drop out water from the back.

Make sense? I want you to practice this with your hands on your hips, going back and forth and finding that neutral (think level bowl) while you are breathing. It might feel sticky and awkward for you, but the more we can practice this and be aware of how your positioning is, the better it will make you feel!

For another visual, during pregnancy, I want you to imagine a string going from your ankle bone up to your knee, going up through your hip bone, up to your shoulders, up through your neck, and coming out the top of your head. Pretend you're pulling up on that string, and that is going to help keep all of your body parts in alignment with a neutral pelvis.

Another important aspect of keeping a neutral pelvis in alignment is not flaring your rib cage out, which can be challenging during the late stages of pregnancy. Being aware of this throughout your pregnancy will continue to help you keep your body in alignment and support your recovery during the postpartum phase.

Let's review:

- Posture for everyday life during pregnancy is often overlooked as a cause of aches and pains.
- Proper posture can reduce pressure on your pelvic floor, your pressure system, and reduce symptoms of a diastasis.
- Maintaining an awareness of proper posture, strength, and alignment will provide the least amount of pain and pressure on your low back, shoulders, and neck.

Coning or doming during pregnancy

During pregnancy, specifically during the second and third trimesters, you may notice coning in your abdomen even as you get out of bed in the morning, off the couch, or during a specific forward-facing movement. If you go back to those images of your anatomy, you will notice that the top layer of your core muscles, the rectus abdominis, is held together down your midline by a thick layer of fascia. Our bodies were wonderfully created this way so our abdomen could expand and grow a small human!

If you see this happening, it is your body's way of telling you, your core pressure is not being regulated. This is why it is important to roll to your side to get out of bed in the morning or be aware of doing that belly pump as you shift around so you are protecting your fascia and inner core muscles. If you see it while doing a plank, push-ups, or another movement in your exercise, your body is telling you the same thing; your pressure is not regulated. This is why it is important to avoid moves that will put excess pressure on your core in this way and why understanding how to control your internal pressure system is a must. As you practice rehabbing your core after the baby, you continue to progress in movements that will put pressure on your core. Only continue with said movements when no coning or doming is present.

The importance of weight-training/weight-bearing movement throughout pregnancy

I wanted to plug this in here because it's something I wish someone had told me during my first pregnancy. As we age, we lose muscle mass; I'm talking 3 percent of muscle each year once we hit our thirties. This is why around this time, many of us start to notice body composition changes, not fitting into our clothes, as well and things just start to sit differently on our bodies.

A very important part of understanding functional fitness is understanding that weight training is needed to keep your muscles growing—weight training in the form of lifting weights or doing weight-bearing movements, such as Pilates or barre. However, here is the catch: During pregnancy, you are not in a growth period. You are in a maintenance period. Due to hormonal changes and that you are growing a small human (or multiples), muscle gains are extremely hard to do.

Muscle gains only take place if they are going through hypertrophy, which is when your muscle meets complete failure with a combination of sets and reps. This is something that is very individual to each person based on their goals. During pregnancy and the initial postpartum phase, we are not focusing on muscle hypertrophy. Our bodies need movement during pregnancy and postpartum, but it looks much different from movement outside of the perinatal season.

The importance of focusing on functional fitness moves throughout pregnancy is to support your posture, gain stability throughout your body, and stay strong enough to meet the demands of your pregnancy and new motherhood phase. This is where many women who become pregnant or looking to become pregnant are overwhelmed in the pregnancy fitness industry. Typically, today you only see pregnant moms (when searching the Internet) who are extremely ripped, stating claims that they only gained X amount of weight during pregnancy or are in the gym, lifting heavy weights.

This is fantastic for them, but this is not our average mom. Many of us have never been to a gym, let alone want to start now that we are pregnant, especially during that first trimester, which is why focusing on lower-impact movements you can do throughout your day is much more achievable.

With this being said, your pregnancy workouts should not be exhausting. Your muscles can and should feel fatigued, but they should be giving you energy to get through the rest of your day. If they are depleting you, it could be because you are focusing too much on a gaining muscle program, and looking for something less intense would be beneficial. The goal of workouts during pregnancy are to stay active, build stamina, and keep your muscle memory moving so you have strength in the areas you need it.

I recommend that during pregnancy, you focus on walking, your everyday movements focusing on functional body mechanics, and doing some form of Pilates and barre geared toward pregnant women. This type of movement is not as stress inducing on the body, and there is a strong focus of proper core activation in all the moves. In 2016, the ACOG began to recommend modified Pilates as a preferred form of movement for pregnant women due to the benefits of stability, core, and posture work that is achieved through this practice. Barre is also a program that is rooted in physical therapy moves and really focuses on building your stabilizing muscles, which, as I've mentioned many times, is so very important for your body throughout pregnancy. Of course, every pregnancy is different; every individual is different. If there is another form of movement that fills you, by all means, do that. Just remember to add in functional movement relating to your core four and strengthen those stabilizing muscles.

Functional fitness

Functional fitness truly is understanding how your body works, what muscles become affected during pregnancy, and how to keep those muscles in top-functioning shape so you can:

1. Prepare for your labor and birth
2. Prepare for the season of motherhood
3. Reduce pain in your body
4. Heal and recover quicker
5. Gain back your energy

How many times a day do you go to sit on the toilet? Every time you do that, you're doing a squat. How many times a day do you pick up a toddler (or will be lifting a newborn baby who weighs 6–9 lbs.), lifting that car seat, carrying those bags? As your baby is growing in your belly, you are carrying the extra weight that comes with that, so it only makes sense to focus on strength moves that support stability so you can feel strong and reduce aches and pains.

The truth is, moms are in a constant state of motion: lifting, pulling, pushing, and twisting. Functional fitness allows you to move better in these moves so you can be strong for your children, feel strong, and reduce common aches, pains, and misalignments.

When you understand how your body works—the deep core, correct engagement—it makes moving in your everyday movements that much easier. This will only benefit you for decades to come and allow you to live a healthy fulfilling life no matter what obstacle may come your way.

When you understand your body and how to connect to your deep core, you can utilize that belly pump as you pick your kiddo off the floor, bend over the bathtub, pick up that laundry basket, grocery bag, or car seat. Heck, you can literally do squats when you use the toilet. Adding in functional pregnancy training can be as simple as that. I share a simple plan you can incorporate into your busy day in the back of this book. Fitness in this season of pregnancy is so much more than it looks; it's all about how to keep strong, feel good, prepare your body for labor and birth, and to reduce daily aches and pains.

Cardio during pregnancy
HIIT or walking or running? What cardio is best?

Before I share what cardio is best for pregnancy and postpartum, let's first define what HIIT and HIT mean and what walking or LISS means because these are thrown all around the Internet today, and everyone will claim one is better than the other.

HIIT means high intensity interval training at a max effort of nine to ten. You do a series of movements or running or on the bike of max effort for a short time combined with short periods of rest so your heart rate goes up and then down throughout the moves. HIIT is good for your cardiovascular system. However, due to the nature of how stressful it can be for your body, it is best to modify the movement to a lower intensity if you choose to do this throughout your pregnancy. That is where high intensity training (HIT) comes in. HIT is more of a moderate effort, with seven or eight max effort, which is recommended for pregnancy. If you were previously doing HIIT prepregnancy and want to continue with something similar, replace it with HIT. During pregnancy, your heart expands to allow more blood flow due to the demands of growing another human, so you will become shorter of breath. Throughout pregnancy, it is best to do the talk test during moves. You should still be able to have a breathy conversation. If doing moves leave you completely breathless, this would be a sign to modify the movement.

The *benefits of HIIT* and HIT are the following: burns many calories in a short period of time; metabolic rate is higher for the entire day, increasing more fat burn; reduces heart and blood pressure; increases oxygen.

LISS, or low-intensity steady state cardio, is a steady state of any form of cardio: walking, jogging, biking, swimming. It is enough to get your heart rate up but slow enough where you can still have a conversation.

Benefits of LISS are improved blood flow, reduced stress, lowers risk of heart disease, and improved brain function. It supports fat burning and fat loss.

Intense moves, such as burpees, jumping jacks, and jump squats during pregnancy are going to feel really hard especially later in your pregnancy. Your blood volume increases, which makes it feel harder to breathe (that feeling of being out of breath even when talking!). In the earlier stages of pregnancy, HIT cycling is a great low-impact form to keep your heart conditioned, or alternating fast-and-slow-interval walking is another great choice. In the later stages of pregnancy or at any point, LISS is excellent and still prepares you for the endurance of labor and birth.

Walking daily for ten to thirty minutes during pregnancy is such a wonderful way to prepare your body for labor, birth, and the demands of motherhood, but it is often overlooked. Walking is such a great choice for those who are just beginning or feeling overwhelmed by doing other intense programs.

Adding in a ten- to thirty-minute walk daily is excellent for your health, and it's the perfect exercise to begin once you have a baby. I cannot recommend walking enough!

A quick note about running during pregnancy because it is a highly searched question from newly pregnant mothers, specifically those who are running while they find out they are pregnant: Running during pregnancy is very personal to the individual. If you are an athlete, who has consistently trained in running for years, you will most likely run more than the average pregnant mother, and that is okay. The important thing to remember when running pregnant is that the added weight to your pelvic floor grows as your baby grows. Typically, most moms feel fine running into their second trimester. It is recommended that you slowly switch to walking/fast walking by twenty weeks due to the increased weight on your pelvic floor. Running is not something you want to begin as a newly pregnant mother. There is increased risk for injury. And as noted above, walking is just as beneficial!

Ideally, as a runner, you need to do what is most comfortable for you. You might stop sooner than your second trimester, and that is okay. It does not make you less than or weak or anything else you might tell yourself. Maybe you run longer because it feels good, and that is okay too. The health of your pelvic floor is really important, so don't run if it hurts! Running into your third trimester of pregnancy, keep in mind, you are not setting time goals. Running during pregnancy is a season, so take it as a season of eliminating PRs, race times, and the like.

Preparing for birth

Now let's get to the good part: preparing for your birth! A very important piece about birth prep is that you need to understand and put into practice the six foundations discussed earlier to train your body so you can be ready for your dream birth. There is zero judgment here. You can be planning a natural (all birth is natural), unmedicated birth; epidural birth; home birth; or hospital birth, I won't tell you otherwise because it is *your* birth. We *all* have an image of what this might look like.

Regardless of your plan, understand that the actual outcome of your birth may not go as you planned. However, controlling how you prepare is only going to increase your ability to handle these changes as they come. Following the guidelines I have listed for you in this book is going to set you up for success. Let's be honest, birth is the scary part of being pregnant, especially if this is your first baby. Everyone will tell you the horror stories, what to do, and what not to. It is important to channel your energy to a positive place throughout your pregnancy, so it is okay for you to tell others that you are only keeping positive thoughts about this. If you are here reading this, you are already so far ahead in understanding how your body works. This is going to help you so much in your birth preparation.

Preparing your body for labor and birth takes the duration of the time you're pregnant, but if you're a month away from having a baby and just reading this, it is never too late to learn this information and put it into practice.

Women have been birthing babies since the beginning of time. It is a natural process, and God designed you for this. You are capable of doing this hard thing. It is a challenge, but you are so capable of achieving this great feat. Labor and birth are trauma to your body, which is why it is important to do all of this preparation work so you are confident as you enter the labor, birth, and recovery stage.

Here is what you need to do to begin your birth prep plan:

- Understand functional body mechanics
- Daily walking
- Connect to your deep core (learn the belly pump).
- Labor training exercises and meditations
- Hiring a doula or labor support is a great option to look into.

As you continue to read this book, everything here is listed out and explained. So by the time you are done reading this book, you will know the exact steps to prepare your body for the demands of labor, birth, and motherhood. Let's be honest, motherhood is the hardest part after you birth your baby. (And I don't have a book for that part yet. Ha!)

Birth center options

There are several options that you can take in preparation on where you will actually have your baby. Where you are located could limit your options of what is available, but it is always good to do a search and see what comes up in your area. You have the option to go the traditional hospital route. Some hospitals offer midwife or doula support as part of their care. You can opt to see just a midwife and give birth at home or a birth center. A birth center is not a hospital and will provide more of a hands-off approach in your labor and delivery. You can also hire a doula for labor and delivery support in the hospital or any other setting that you choose. There is no right or wrong place to give birth; you have to go where you feel the most supported and comfortable.

Labor training, meditation, and affirmation exercises

Labor training exercises are very specific exercise circuits to prepare your body for labor. (There is a guide for you in the back of this book.) You should do a labor-training workout at least one to three times a week. They are specific because they have you in a work/rest combination that mimics the flow of contractions. For example, when you first begin labor training, you will begin with a forty-five-second workout period with a one-minute rest. You will complete one movement at a fast pace for those forty-five seconds to mimic the contraction, while the rest phase is to mimic the actual rest that comes between a contraction.

The movement that you do during this forty-five-second work period could be walking at a fast pace, cycling, or doing a specific strengthening movement to get your heart rate up. During the one-minute rest period, you would want to stop the movement, focus on your breathing, and repeat those positive affirmations to yourself. You can practice mindfulness and positive affirmations at any point in your pregnancy; however, doing it during the labor training is the best practice because when a movement feels hard, you want to tell yourself "I can do this!"

Labor (and motherhood) is not only physical but a challenge mentally. Our thoughts have a very, very powerful effect on our outcomes and mostly how we *feel* about those outcomes. Many of us may not even be aware of the thoughts that go through our head daily, and taking an effort to be aware of them and to focus on positive ones is a very powerful practice.

Labor is a big challenging event. I am not going to sugarcoat it and tell you it is going to be easy, but I am here to tell you that without a doubt, you can do it, and you have to start telling yourself that! Here is a list of birth affirmations that are commonly used. Please be sure to adapt them to fit your needs best.

These affirmations should be repeated daily, even written daily (be sure to check out the *Daily Take Five Journal* and the *Pregnancy Fitness Journal* I wrote, available on Amazon). Say them in your workouts when it gets hard. Congratulate yourself when you have completed some reps or when you completed something that was hard.

- I am strong.
- I am capable.
- I am birthing this baby exactly how I am supposed to be.
- I breathe my baby down with each contraction.
- I will focus on my breath with each contraction.
- I am getting closer to meeting my baby.
- Each contraction is a wave that I can breathe through.
- I can do this.
- My baby and I are working together.
- My body is strong and capable.
- My body and my baby are working together.
- I release the fear of judgment in my birth choices.
- Regardless of my birth outcome, I know my body is strong.

A large part of having a successful birth is to understand labor positioning and birthing positions that support your body design. Did you know that women started birthing on their backs centuries ago when a king wanted to watch his wife give birth?

For some reason, over time, this is what we commonly see in the media, mothers giving birth on their backs despite the fact there is clear evidence that it is not a good position. The American College of Obstetricians and Gynecologists (ACOG) actually states that *"there is little evidence that any one position is best. Moreover, the traditional supine position during labor has known adverse effects, such as supine hypotension and more frequent fetal heart rate decelerations. Therefore, for most women, no one position needs to be mandated or proscribed."*

Ya'll, the organization that does research on women during pregnancy, birth, and the postpartum phase literally is saying that lying supine has negative effects during birth, yet this continues to be what the majority of doctors "prescribe." For one, as you lay on your back, it constricts the pelvic opening, and you are lying on your aorta, which causes the lack of blood flow and oxygen to your baby.

Standing in an upright position allows natural gravity to help the baby out, along with allowing our pelvic floor and bone structure to support the widest opening. Also, when you're upright, the uterus can contract more strongly and efficiently, helping get the baby in a better position to pass through the pelvis. There has been MRI evidence to show that the outlet of your pelvis actually becomes wider if you're squatting or kneeling. There is research that has found that upright birthing positions increase a mother's satisfaction and lead to a more positive birth experience. Some birth positions that are helpful to try out:

- Hands and knees
- Squatting
- Kneeling while leaning off a bed/chair
- Kneeling
- Sitting on a toilet (positioning is optimal for opening your pelvic floor)
- Side lying (especially helpful for those who choose an epidural)

- Having your knees close together and your feet farther apart in any of the above positions really opens the pelvis.

Despite this information and potential benefits, most people giving birth in the US hospitals report giving birth on their backs or in a semisitting position where they lay in bed with the head of the bed raised up. A very small minority give birth in other positions. In an interview with a midwife, she stated that the majority of her clients spontaneously give birth on their hands and knees. I would like to put a note in here that this is a very important topic to discuss with your provider. Many times, women give birth on their back because it is the most convenient position for the provider and seems to be the status quo. Some providers are going to be more open to this than others, which is why it is *so* important to discuss this topic. We can all be adults in these situations, and I want to empower you to be assertive in how you bring up this topic. Feel free to remind your provider of those findings on ACOG about birth positions. Remember that *you* are the one giving birth. You have every right to be in the position that best *serves you and your body*, not your provider. It can feel challenging to have this discussion, so be sure to have the support of your partner and express to your provider that it would make you feel comfortable knowing you might be in a different position than your back to birth. I personally was on all fours for all but my last birth because that is what felt most comfortable for my body, and my last birth was the most difficult for me!

There are countless studies to back up the fact that upright positions not only have a more positive effect on labor but that the number of hours of labor are decreased, and less interventions are needed. There is limited data on birthing upright with the use of an epidural. But one study that took place in Sweden had over five hundred mothers who had an epidural give birth in a squatting position over a squat toilet, and these all had positive outcomes.

The last thing I want to note about laboring is that motion is lotion. The more that you can move, change positions, walk, even sit over the toilet to support your contractions is the best way to help the baby move down and out. During the later weeks of pregnancy, thirty-five weeks and beyond, it is important to sit on a birth ball; sit upright; sit on your knees, leaning on a birth ball or couch and taking walks. (The seemingly small act of putting one foot in front of the other opens up our pelvis to prepare for baby is so underrated!) Even if you choose to have an epidural, you can move—positioning, side lying specifically to create opening and movement for yourself while pushing the baby out. Practicing some of these moves and doing pelvic floor relaxation are helpful as you get closer to your due date.

Another important fact to supporting a relaxed pelvic floor during the labor stage is to have a relaxed face and jaw. These muscles are directly related to our pelvic floor. If or when you clench your jaw or face, your pelvic floor will simultaneously clench. As contractions become more intense, making an open-mouthed moan (almost like a yoga chant) is extremely beneficial in keeping your pelvic floor open and helping you get through the intensity of the contraction. Most women do not go through a natural childbirth without making sounds of some sort. This is natural, and it is important to let your body do what it needs to do through this process. I remember going through my first labor; I thought to myself, *Holy moly, I literally sound like a cow.* But my nurse was *amazing* and continued to tell me that was the best way to work through those contractions. And by golly, it was really helpful, to say the least!

Doula support

Another support during labor would be to hire a doula. These are individuals who are trained in birthing techniques with the least number of interventions possible. It is helpful to review your birth wishes with them and have this extra support during the labor and birth period. They know how to position, move, massage, and do other simple techniques to support you in having a positive, empowering birth experience. Depending on what state or country you are in, you should be able to do a local search to find doula support near you.

Pelvic floor relaxation

When you are about thirty weeks pregnant, you will want to begin what we call pelvic-floor relaxation. As you perform your belly pump, you will *not* bring your pelvic floor up as you tighten your TVA. You will relax it, allowing it to open as you birth your baby down breath by breath. This is best practiced while sitting on a birthing ball, on a yoga block, in a child's pose, while kneeling over your bed, or sitting on the toilet. Any of those positions I mentioned before to get your body into that motion and practice when the contractions come. You can do this, friend, and I am cheering for you!

Pregnancy nutrition

We are not going to complicate nutrition during pregnancy any more than we have too. We are *bombarded* with information overload about diets, nutrition, weight loss, and the like so much that you probably don't even know what the heck to do about it. I'm going to stick to the facts here so you have a simple plan moving forward.

Your first trimester might leave you feeling under the radar, and food will most likely be the last thing you think of. Toast, crackers, rice, noodles might be the only thing you are consuming, and that is okay. This is not the time to put any pressure or expectations on yourself about a plan. The thought of eating any vegetable might make you want to hurl; I get it. During the first trimester, your body is going into overdrive to grow little junior, and you just need to let it run its course.

One thing that is helpful during this time is to eat every few hours, drink a lot of water, and do your best to eat protein at each meal/snack. Eating enough protein will lessen your feelings of being nauseous and stabilize your blood sugars. It's a period of time that will not last forever, so don't be too concerned that you aren't eating all the whole foods. You can only do your best!

Unfortunately, society has totally skewed our view on nutrition. As you read this, I want you to wipe away any misconceptions you may have had about food. That carbs are bad, low fat is best, more cardio, etc. Toss that out the window, take it way back, and start with food as fuel. You are going to focus on food as fuel for you and your baby! The first thing you need to understand are whole foods and macronutrients, so let's dive in.

What are whole foods?

Whole food is any food that comes from the ground or has a mother, the foods that God created for our bodies to function best from—for example, chicken, fish, red meat, eggs, all fruits and vegetables, legumes, nuts, seeds. This does not mean you should not eat sliced bread but focus on the bread that is made with fresh flour and has the least amount of ingredients and preservatives.

Honestly, y'all, our bodies were designed to eat food in its most natural state, and that overall will have the largest impact on how you feel, your energy, the amount of excess weight you gain, and so forth. Many of us automatically think, *I have to exercise a lot to not gain weight*, when in reality, nutrition makes up 90 percent of our efforts of weight gain or weight loss. I will discuss more about weight loss in the postpartum section. You do not want to focus on weight loss during pregnancy; your main focus should be eating quality nutrients to fuel yourself and your baby.

What are macronutrients?

Macronutrients are your fats, carbs, and proteins, literally that simple. I am going to break down what each macronutrient is, why it is important, and give you examples of what a whole food is in each macronutrient.

Fats

Fat is a critical part of our diet, and undereating this macronutrient has negative effects on your body. When you ingest the proper amount of healthy fats in your diet, you support your metabolism, immunity, hormones, and body composition. Fat does not make you fat. Your body was designed to eat fats, and not eating enough of the proper amount causes more harm than good.

Healthy fats include the following:

- Avocado
- Olive oil
- Coconut oil
- Nuts
- Fat from salmon, grass-fed meat, eggs
- Due to the high omega three fatty acids in salmon, this is one thing you should try to eat one to two times a week while pregnant.

Carbohydrates

Carbohydrates are molecules composed of carbon, oxygen, and hydrogen. Carbohydrates are important nutrients for energy and for building cells in the body. Carbohydrates are your primary source for fuel for organs and muscles. They fuel your workouts, increase energy levels, and trigger the release of insulin. Whole food carbohydrates support thyroid function, lean muscle mass, and even our gut health.

Whole food carbohydrates include the following:

- Sweet potatoes and white potatoes
- Rice, brown rice, bulgur
- Oats, steel cut oats, barley
- Legumes
- Fruit!

Protein

Protein is a very important macronutrient as it is literally needed for every growth process, including growing your baby and keeping lean muscle mass for you. Proteins are naturally occurring compounds that are used for the growth and repair in the body and to build cells and tissues. Your muscle tissue contains a lot of protein. It keeps you strong and makes your bones last. It is an extremely important macronutrient to consume the right amount during pregnancy.

Your body really needs protein as it is the building block to giving you energy and helps your growing baby develop adequately. Most of us do not *eat enough*. Especially for women, we tend to have this thought process of less is more. Less will make me thinner or keep me thinner throughout pregnancy. There is a study that I am taking part in actually, so the results are not out yet but pertaining to weight gain during pregnancy and postpartum. One of the questions asked was, Does or did the weight gain have a negative impact on your postpartum journey? And the resounding *yes* on all the surveys was shocking to me. This is obviously a challenge that needs to be discussed with perinatal women, and I am going to show you a simple way to help you with this by learning how to build a plate so that you can feel confident in how you fuel your body during pregnancy and can reduce excess weight gain.

Whole food proteins:

- Eggs or egg white
- Ground beef and other cuts of quality meat
- Chicken
- White fish
- Salmon
- Pork

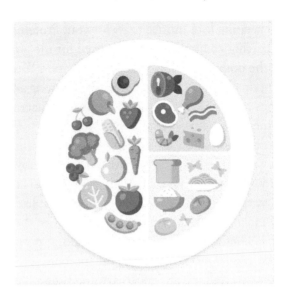

How to build a plate

Americans really do overthink their diets, and it's not our fault; it's the system. So again, just wipe away any weird thing you've ever heard before, and start fresh with this perspective!

Every time you eat, you want to focus on your plate being filled with one-half vegetables, one-fourth starches/carbohydrates (about half a cup), one-fourth protein (the size of your palm), and about two to three tablespoons (two thumbs worth) of healthy fats at each meal. This can be in the form of the protein you are having, a salad dressing with quality olive oil, or some nuts on top of your salad. There is no diet approach that works for everyone, but what you need to focus on is eating whole foods and in those portion sizes the best you can. Keep focusing on that, and just see what happens. Ideally focusing on 20–30g of protein at each meal will make a large difference in your energy and how you feel and support your strength as well as for your growing baby.

Overall, during pregnancy, you only need about three hundred to four hundred extra calories in the second and third trimesters, closer to four hundred or so during the later stages of your third trimester. I don't like to focus so much on counting calories as it's very vague. If you focus on building your plate in the way I shared, eating three meals and two snacks, adding in a third snack in your third trimester, this should leave you feeling energized and strong. During your third trimester, you have very little room for food (thanks, baby!), so focusing on several small meals a day usually is what works best. So make sure you are prepared for this.

Here are some great snack ideas, remembering to keep them in these portions.

Pregnancy snack ideas:

- Mixed nuts (raisins, almonds, pistachios, walnuts, pecans)
- Apple with a cheese stick or some nut butter (think only two thumbs worth!)
- Sliced veggies with hummus
- Hard-boiled eggs
- Rice cakes topped with nut butter, or avocado and sliced turkey (nitrate-free)
- Deli turkey (nitrate-free) rolled up with a pickle or in a lettuce leaf
- Beef stick or beef jerky
- Smoothie with protein powder or collagen powder (*needed brand*), frozen fruit, and spinach/kale/cauliflower
- Yogurt smoothie bowl with drizzle of maple syrup, 1 tsp. dark chocolate chips
- Avocado toast with tomato
- Chia seed pudding

Sugar and sweets during pregnancy. So many of us have the all-or-nothing mindset. We think we have to eat nothing but the veggies and chicken to reach our goals, but this usually sets us up for failure. If you want one piece of dark chocolate each night as you have your cup of tea, do that. If you prefer ice cream or cake, do that, but limit it to one to two times a week, and eat a serving size.

As far as setting yourself up for success, don't overthink it. Pick a few things you enjoy for breakfast and just keep rotating them. For lunch, stick to a large, leafy green salad with a quality protein source. For dinner, there are so many quick recipes out there for one-pot meals, a meal that has protein, carbs, and vegetables. It really is as simple as that. Eating enough protein is going to be the most beneficial for you as this is the building block of growing your baby. For reference, I have a list on my fridge of what I will feed my children for breakfast every day (and myself). We rotate through the same thing each week. I make the *same thing* every day for breakfast: eggs and mushrooms or any leftover veggie that is already cooked from the night before. If you have minimal time in the morning, make a large egg bake with veggies for the week so all you need to do is grab and reheat. Throw it on a slice of whole wheat bread, and you have a quick egg sandwich. Be sure to head to my blog www.kaitlinspano.co and join the community, where I send weekly recipes that are quick, healthy, and don't break the bank. As a homeschooling family, business owner, and mom of five young children, I spend about 75 percent of my day making meals for my children and myself. The other 25 percent is spent thinking about what meals to make. *Ha!*

Moral of healthy nutrition habits: Stick to whole foods, balance each plate with the plate-it method, enjoy a few treats a few times a week, and make a weekly plan so you know what to expect. It is that simple! Another key point that is important for you to understand is that dairy-free, paleo, vegan, vegetarian, pescetarian, keto diets, etc. are just a preferred eating style. One is not better over the other. Again, stick to eating whole foods and foods that make you feel good! Focus on how food makes you feel, and this awareness is what should fuel what to eat versus what you might not choose.

In the postpartum section, I review macronutrients for breastfeeding and navigating weight loss after baby.

Miscarriage and infant loss

This is not an enjoyable topic or exciting to read about, but it is the reality for many women. One in four women will experience a miscarriage or infant loss in their life. It is important to understand that everyone who experiences this type of loss come from all walks of life and you are allowed to feel what you feel. It affects everyone differently, and your feelings are valid. I have experienced a miscarriage myself and have had several friends who have all walked paths of miscarriage, stillbirth, and infant loss.

I am going to share the different types of miscarriages that women experience, as well as resources that could be of use to you or someone else you know. It is also important to understand that if you go through a miscarriage or infant loss, you are not alone and have the right to ask for support while having resources to support you through this difficult time. Please note the resource page for miscarriage and stillbirth at the end of this book.

There are several types of miscarriage: *threatened, inevitable, complete, incomplete, or missed.* Other types of pregnancy loss include an ectopic pregnancy, molar pregnancy, and a blighted ovum. These are all terms that your provider may have to discuss with you, so I'm going to give the definition of each, then I will go into some common questions about miscarriage and finally how to care for yourself if this is something that you end up having to experience.

Miscarriage is the expulsion of a fetus from the womb before it can survive independently, especially spontaneously or as the result of accident.

Early pregnancy loss

The loss of a pregnancy before thirteen weeks may also be referred to as a spontaneous abortion. The American College of Obstetricians and Gynecologists (ACOG) estimates, it is the most common form of pregnancy loss. It is estimated that as many as 26 percent of all pregnancies end in miscarriage and up to 10 percent of clinically recognized pregnancies. Moreover, 80 percent of early pregnancy loss occurs in the first trimester. The risk of miscarriage decreases after twelve weeks gestation.

Threatened miscarriage

Threatened miscarriage is bleeding from the vagina and symptoms that may mean a higher risk of miscarriage. It happens during the first three months (or twenty weeks) of pregnancy. Not everyone who has bleeding in early pregnancy will miscarry.

Inevitable miscarriage

It refers to the presence of bleeding in the first trimester of pregnancy. Most often, the tissues and fetus are not expelled, and intracervical contents may be present at the time of examination. A sac may be seen low within the uterus, and progressive migration of the same may be demonstrated on serial scans.

Essentially, a threatened miscarriage progresses to an inevitable miscarriage if cervical dilatation occurs. Once tissue has passed through the cervix, this will then be termed an incomplete miscarriage, and ultimately a complete miscarriage.

Complete miscarriage is defined as a cessation of vaginal bleeding with no evidence of retained products of conception or a gestation sac in a woman who previously had an ultrasound confirmed intrauterine pregnancy.

Incomplete miscarriage is a term given to miscarriage where some of the tissue or fetus are retained in the uterus.

Missed miscarriage, a missed miscarriage, sometimes termed a missed abortion, is a situation when there is a non-viable fetus within the uterus, without symptoms of a miscarriage.

Ectopic pregnancy refers to the implantation of a fertilized ovum outside of the uterine cavity.

Anembryonic pregnancy is a form of a failed early pregnancy, where a gestational sac develops, but the embryo does not form.

Molar pregnancy is one of the common complications of gestation and estimated to occur in one of every one thousand to two thousand pregnancies. These moles can occur in a pregnant woman of any age, but the rate of occurrence is higher in pregnant women in their teens or between the ages of forty to fifty years.

Stillbirth

Stillbirth is when a fetus dies in the uterus after twenty weeks of pregnancy. A stillbirth can happen during labor and birth, and there really is not a clear explanation of why these occur. There are some possible causes, such as genetic defect, growth problems from the placenta, umbilical cord, infections or medical condition from the mother, or a complication that arose during labor and delivery.

Stillbirth is a profoundly painful event for those affected by it. Grief is a normal, natural response, and it is important to mourn your loss for as long as you need. It is important to remember that each parent/family grieves in a different way. Talking with your partner or another person you trust about what you are feeling and experiencing is helpful. Some women also find it helpful to talk with others who have gone through this. Please refer to the resources at the end of this book for support organizations.

What causes a miscarriage?

There is not a specific cause of why a miscarriage may happen. However, over half of miscarriages happen when the embryo does not develop properly. This is often due to an abnormal number of chromosomes. If an egg or sperm has too little or too many chromosomes, the fetus will result in an abnormal amount which can also lead to miscarriage.

A miscarriage is not a woman's fault, so don't ever, ever blame yourself. It is usually a random event, and there has been zero research to back up any type of exercise or activity that could cause a miscarriage.

Symptoms

Bleeding from the vagina is the most common symptom of a miscarriage. Not all spotting will result in a miscarriage; however, if you happen to have bleeding or spotting, contact your doctor right away. Another sign of a miscarriage is feeling a gush, even if there is no blood, or passing tissue. If you experience either of these things, it is important to contact your doctor.

Some women begin early labor during a miscarriage and experience a typical labor and delivery, even though the baby is too small.

Let it be noted that *no question or concern* is too small to contact your doctor! They are there for you, and it is better to ask them anything you may be experiencing instead of searching for it on Google.

Treatment

After a miscarriage, some tissue may be left in the uterus, and this is what we refer to as an incomplete miscarriage.

Treatment is very individual to the person and the situation and how many weeks your baby was. If you do not show any sign of infection, you can wait and pass the tissue naturally as your body will do this on its own. This can be hard because there is no timeline, everybody and every body is different, and it can be hard to wait for this to happen.

There is medication that you can take to help expel the tissue faster, if that feels like a better solution for you. Surgery is another option and may be needed if your baby is beyond twenty weeks. A dilation and curettage (D&C) is one surgery option where they dilate your cervix and remove all the tissue from your uterus.

The other form of surgery, which is less common, is a vacuum aspiration in which they suck all the contents out of your uterus.

Recovery

Recovery is necessary after a miscarriage, yet many women don't take this time because they downplay the event. However, just as birth is trauma to your body, so is a miscarriage. You will experience bleeding after a miscarriage, just as you do after the birth of your baby. Bleeding time varies, but the reason you bleed after a birth is because your placenta leaves a hole in your uterus. This needs time to heal, which is why rest is important.

Talk with your provider about trying to conceive again, but usually it is dependent on how you feel about the situation and when you are ready.

Losing a pregnancy can cause grief and sadness. For many women, it takes longer to heal emotionally than physically. It is important to ask for help, reach out to support groups, and talk to your partner or reach out to a therapist to help you process this information. There is no right way or wrong way to grieve a miscarriage, and your feelings are valid.

Other pregnancy conditions

There are several pregnancy conditions that could come up for you as you navigate pregnancy, such as the following:

- Gestational diabetes
- Preeclampsia
- High blood pressure
- Hyperemesis gravidarum
- Placenta previa
- Preterm labor
- Multiple pregnancy

These are some of the more common (though not common) pregnancy conditions that you may encounter. It is important to follow the guidance of your obstetrician or midwife regarding your condition and follow the care plan that you and your provider work together to create so that you feel comfortable and cared for as you navigate your pregnancy.

Some conditions may force you to be on bed rest. The amazing thing is that you can *still* focus on your breathing, activating your core four, affirmations, and gentle movements while restraining yourself from other activities. This will keep your stress levels down and allow you to focus on things *you can control* while so many others are out of your control.

The perfect birth

Now, I do want to be realistic with you: The perfect birth does not exist. Women tend to judge each other about the way other women give birth or their circumstances. No birth is better than another; you have to do what you are most comfortable with. You do not have to have a home birth to have a hands-off, intervention-free birth. This can also happen in the hospital; you just have to communicate with your providers and birth team so they know what your expectations are. We can do all the work we can, read our affirmations, and make the birth plan; yet life still happens, and unexpected things take place. Maybe it was so much harder than you anticipated, maybe the baby was in the wrong position despite your efforts, maybe your epidural failed or you decided you needed one because you were into hour 30 and you needed to rest. Despite our best efforts, unexpected events can still happen and can leave us with feelings of failure or shame.

Does this make you a failure? *No.* It makes you human, regardless of how your birth ended. You are strong; you are amazing; you brought life into the world. The worst thing we can do as women is hold onto those expectations that we failed. The thoughts we hold in our head can be devastating for our mental health, so be sure to journal or talk about what you enjoyed and what you didn't, what happened as planned or what did not. God does not make mistakes. Regardless of our plan, God has already laid one out for us. We need to trust in that. Preparing our bodies and minds is extremely important and will benefit you throughout your motherhood years. Until it happens, until that moment, think positive thoughts. Connect to your powerhouse, and trust that God has great things planned for you and your little one regardless of the outcome.

Part 3

Postpartum Recovery and Rehab

Here you are, on the other side of pregnancy! You did it. See, I knew you could. Regardless of how your birth went, it is important to take time to heal, rehab, and restore your body. You literally completed the marathon of pregnancy, and now you are preparing for the never-ending marathon of motherhood. New research has *finally* come out that postpartum recovery, from a cellular and biomechanical level, can take anywhere from two to seven years. So do not feel pressured to be somewhere you are not based on the media or other outside sources.

This section is not a weight-loss program, a high-intensity fitness program, or a diet for you to get your body back. Your body never left you, and my goodness, look at what it grew for you!

I understand that living in your postpartum body can feel awkward, hard, and if this is your first time here, it can feel really isolating and lonely. Whatever you are feeling at this point in time, know that your feelings are valid! Postpartum hits differently for everyone, and it's important to lean into what you need while still creating space for *you*. You are a mother now, but that does not define you completely; it is now just a part of you.

What this section will provide for you is a system that will allow you space to heal, restore, and replenish so that you can get back to a daily routine that feels good for *you. Your body, your routine.*

So with that being said, we will review as follows:

1. Postpartum body mechanics
2. Vaginal birth recovery
3. Cesarean birth recovery
4. Postpartum depletion
5. Postpartum nutrition
6. Rehab, restore, and replenish

The benefits of a postpartum healing program go beyond any type of aesthetics that we, the moms, are over-exposed too as soon as we have a baby. We are not here to get our body back. (It never left!) We are here to bounce forward with our badass body that has now created life and will become stronger than ever before.

Before any new mom begins any sort of postpartum fitness program, they must focus on postpartum rehabili-tation—healing, repairing, and strengthening—from the inside out. During this period of time, a mother should be focused on movement that supports healing of the body, the tissues, and replenishing the depletion that took place during pregnancy.

Postpartum rehab is essential for keeping stress at bay and supporting positive mental health during this incredi-ble yet taxing transition period. Any woman should not feel pressured or less than if you did not begin a fitness routine six weeks after giving birth. Doctors hype us all up at our six-week appointment, saying, "All clear!" I don't know about you, but not once did my doctor give me advice on what to do before that six-week appointment. Well, maybe he told me to monitor my bleeding and any signs of fever, but that's it. Like, hello, we just pushed out (through the door or the sunroof) a 5–8 lbs. small human, and that's all you have to tell me? We so deserve more than this, friend!

The problem with jumping back into a routine too soon is that if you don't take the time to heal, recover, and address postnatal depletion, it will give you adverse effects as time goes on. So let me give you the steps to address these needs so you can feel confident, strong, and energized as a new mom.

With any big body trauma, think knee injury, shoulder surgery, etc., the first prescribed order is physical therapy or rehabilitation. Postpartum mothers are not receiving therapy as a standard protocol, and this needs to end here! There is continued research taking place that a woman's body is *still* repairing itself on a cellular level, a *year* postpartum. For those who are breastfeeding, this will continue beyond the year and post six months beyond when you finish breastfeeding. I mean, y'all, our cells are *everything*!

So, Kaitlin, how and when do I start postpartum rehab? (Hint: It should have started during pregnancy. But if you are just reading this, for postbaby, there is no better time than the present!)

Postpartum body mechanics

Everybody, every body, is different. However, the first thing anyone can do, regardless of how you gave birth, is begin with core breathing and postural alignment as soon as the baby comes out. Go back and touch up on those pregnancy body mechanics if you need to, the same applies for postbaby. Focusing on deep diaphragmatic breathing is the most beneficial thing to do for postbirth to begin the healing process of the tissue, organs, and reducing mental stress. You can start doing this right after you have a baby! And honestly, when your nurse or midwife is pushing on your fundus or when you have to take that first postbaby poop, you'll want to focus on that breath!

Let's review those six foundations as they pertain to your postpartum recovery.

Core four

Your core four is made up of four primary muscles that surround the center of your body, the exact place where we grew that small human (or two or three). Things probably feel sloshy, floppy, smushy in your core area, and that is totally normal! It is normal to look about five to six months pregnant or more after you give birth. Don't let those pictures on the Internet fool you, okay?

Now that you have the understanding of all your core four muscles from the pregnancy section, it is now time to take note of all those muscles again and reconnect and repattern them without the baby in our belly. Keep this in mind, when a baby is born, the placenta that you also birthed has left a small dish plate–sized open wound in your uterus. *This takes time to heal.* So let this be a reminder that it is okay and necessary to take that much-needed rest!

Let's review:

- Now that your baby is out of your abdomen, it is important to reconnect all those inner muscles and heal them.
- Rest and recovery are the first things to healing your core four unit postpartum.

Diaphragmatic breathing

Breathing is the best place to begin your healing process postbaby. Every time you nurse or bottle-feed your baby, this is the best time to relax, focus on that deep rib cage expansion, and release any tension or stress, we are still holding in our body. It also brings more oxygen and blood flow to your nether region to further support healing in our muscles and tissues that were just stretched, yanked, pulled, and maybe cut!

When our babies grow, it literally shifts the insides of our core. Our bladder, our intestines, our stomach all move to make space for baby. Focusing on your breathing will allow these things to slowly start to shift back into place. So much of postpartum healing cannot be seen, which makes it that much harder for us to understand.

Let's review:

- Diaphragmatic breathing is the first step to begin healing postbaby.
- It brings blood flow and oxygen to our injured parts to promote healing.
- It supports the placement of our insides, putting them back into place.

Pelvic floor

Our pelvic floor had a lot of weight on it throughout the duration of our pregnancy. Not only did it have constant tension on it, it also had to stretch about fifty times its size to accommodate the birth of a baby. She did a lot of work, and she needs the proper rest, care, and rehab, just like any other muscle would need if it had trauma. You may have had stitches here or a small tear in your perineum, so it is important to follow your doctor's directions about care on that. You don't want to begin any deep contractions with your pelvic floor until you are about three weeks postpartum. As you focus on your breathing, you can do a few holds and releases just to get the blood flow in this area to support faster healing.

Before you even leave the hospital, or before your midwife leaves, be sure to ask for a referral to see a pelvic floor physical therapist. They will assess your pelvic floor, determine if you have any grade of prolapse, tearing, weakness, or tightness. Even if you go only *once* to see them, it is so empowering and helpful to ask questions and feel heard. Seeing a pelvic floor physical therapist will help your recovery.

Let's review:

- Your pelvic floor stretched fifty times its size during the birth of baby.
- Be sure to ask your OB for a referral to go see a pelvic floor PT so she can assess this muscle.
- Leaking urine or poop after birth is common, but it is *not* normal, and you do not have to suffer in silence.

Transversus abdominis

This muscle was also stretched out to make room for the baby. So again, focusing on that breath, taking some belly pumps while lying down or breastfeeding will not hurt! It is only going to help you reconnect those mind and muscle movements, which will support your healing. Engaging your TVA with your breathing will support and help your uterus contract back down.

Engaging your TVA postbirth provides minor compression to your intestinal tract, which is actually really needed to support healthy digestion and support putting things back into place. Those of you who may suffer from bloating gas issues postbaby, especially those who have given birth via cesarean section, there is a large chance it is because your intestinal tract needs to be stimulated.

You will most likely be feeling cramping from your uterus as it slowly shrinks back down to size. With each baby you have, the cramping tends to be worse, and I can attest to the accuracy of this! When the cramps hit focus on that deep diaphragmatic breathing to help you through, it is only temporary.

Let's review:

- The TVA is the muscle you want to focus on strengthening and healing as it will support your entire kinetic chain.
- Focusing on this deep core muscle will support in healing any separation or diastasis recti that you may be experiencing.

Rectus abdominis

These muscles were stretched out as your abdomen grew. Some of you may be feeling a large gap down your midline or an even larger one around your belly button. The first six weeks after birth, it is normal to have this as your core slowly goes back to life without a baby taking up space. It is important to lean to the side while getting out of bed, off the chair, and activate that active core breath to support equalized pressure in your core unit. I will be discussing diastasis recti later in this section.

Posture

Our posture took a beating throughout pregnancy. Now it is going to continue to be compromised as you will be holding a newborn, nursing or bottle-feeding, holding in one arm and any awkward sleeping positions that may happen. These positions will put tension on our muscles, which can lead to pain, aches, and muscle cramps. Do the best you can to be aware of this, focusing on how forward your head is when feeding the baby, your shoulder placement, and it's really important to focus on that rib placement.

Let's review:

- Being aware of your posture will provide relief in the form of reduced low back, shoulder, and neck pain.

Rib flare

Another important aspect of postpartum rehab is to be aware of your rib cage placement. Many of us have a rib flare situation going on, almost like a bird puffing her chest out. You want to keep your rib cage pulled down and together. Thinking of your rib cage as butterfly wings, be sure to keep them closed and down instead of flared and open, except on that lateral expansion of your breathing. After pregnancy, our bodies become tight in the low back, causing it to arch back into a slight posterior tilt, which causes our ribs to get stuck in that flared bird-with-puffy-chest situation.

This posture takes place because of muscle imbalances and poor posture over time that resulted throughout a pregnancy. This rib flare oftentimes get stuck, meaning the fascia that is all interconnected within your core four is tight and rigid. To start breaking this tight fascia up around the rib cage, one must first start to connect with your breath. Once you begin breathing into your rib cage, this will begin to loosen up the fascia and reduce the muscle tension, which will support the posture, which will support the healing, which will reduce the rib flare. See how that works?

Stretching and foam rolling in certain areas around this rib flare will also support your body in this area. Some stretches that are beneficial are the following:

- Standing side-bend stretch, arms overhead
- Roll on foam roller under armpits to release the lats
- Low back release
- Child's pose

You may begin to feel overwhelmed with the amount of information here, which is normal and okay. I am providing this information to you so you can be aware of it and leave you feeling empowered about your own body. I have several videos on my YouTube channel where I go into more detail about these topics to further support you and empower you on this journey after having your baby.

Vaginal birth recovery

If you had a vaginal birth, all of the foundations pertain to you. As far as recovery, everyone is a bit different in how they feel and also how difficult your labor and actual birth was.

As stated previously, be sure to follow directions if you have stitches or a tear. While in the hospital, it is really helpful to take pain medication as needed and always ask for stool softener! It just helps, and I always recommend taking it the first week that you are home. You will be bleeding, so having pads or using *Thinx* underwear always felt more comfortable for myself. Wear nonrestrictive clothing so you can just be comfortable!

Having a peri bottle is helpful when you use the bathroom (they should give you one in the hospital), and I always had the nurses make a padsicle. They would put an ice pack in a pad and stick that in those nice throwaway undies, and, y'all, it felt so good for those first twenty-four hours postbirth. You can of course do this at any point when you are home as needed. You can make your own and have them ready to go in your freezer for when you need them.

I remember thinking I wanted to take a walk a few days after I had my first son, and I walked for a few minutes and was like, "Okay, I feel weak, exhausted, and my pelvis hurts." Walking is great, but only when you feel ready. But remember, there are no PRs to be chased. Listen to your body.

- Recovery time will fully depend on how invasive your vaginal birth was.
- It is normal to feel sore, tired, and achy after.
- Peri bottle and padsicles are great to support healing those first few weeks.

Cesarean birth recovery

For those who have a cesarean birth, initial recovery will be more intense those first few weeks due to the nature of having a very large incision in your abdomen. Having help lined up to support you while you are home is very important for cesarean recovery. Some of you may not have been planning for a cesarean, so asking your partner to help you set up some at home support will be really helpful.

As always, be sure to follow the guidelines from your doctor on managing the incision and take note of any bleeding, extreme pain, puss, or fever. Lifting anything other than your newborn is off limits. This is where all that breathing practice will come in very helpful for you!

Even though you had a cesarean, you will still bleed vaginally and need to be prepared for this by using pads or disposable diapers or whatever you find most comfortable. You'll want comfortable clothing and loose pants that are not tight on your abdomen. Coughing, laughing, bending, getting out of bed and a chair will also feel challenging as you use your core to do these moves, so move cautiously while doing your best to use your core breathing to support your movements. Having a pillow to cover your incision is helpful when moving out of the bed or coughing.

Staying on top of your medication that is provided will help reduce the pain of your cesarean incision and reduce healing time. Be sure to ask for and take a stool softener while in the hospital and continue to take this while at home. This is going to make that first postsurgery poop so much easier for you.

Stay hydrated, and be sure to empty your bladder every two hours or so. Allow your Steri-Strips to fall off on their own! If one side begins to fall off, you can trim this short until the rest of the strip falls off. A cesarean is a big, invasive surgery; be sure to rest, drink fluids, and give yourself grace. In time you will heal as long as you don't rush it.

How to care for your cesarean scar

Caring for your cesarean birth scar is very important but also very rarely discussed by your provider. Again, each provider, midwife shares different information, but this is something that really needs to be shared to moms who have cesarean surgery.

When your incision is completely healed, you can begin a scar massage to break up scar tissue while bringing feeling back to this area and to reduce adhesions from the inside.

This is usually done at the six-/eight-week mark. Scar massage helps

- Scar tissue from forming in unwanted areas
- Increase blood flow
- Expand flexibility and elasticity
- Lessen pain and sensitivity in surrounding areas
- Reduces thick scar formations
- Prevent infections

You will want to use different grades of material—for example, a cotton ball, a thick piece of cloth with ridges (like a pillow cover), a silky piece of material, and you can also use a gua sha stone to break up scar tissue. You can use vitamin E oil or coconut oil to support the massage of skin.

Using one piece of material at a time, you want to rub around your scar, top and bottom. Go up and down over your scar and also in circles around it. Doing this three to five times a week or even daily, if you can, will support healing of your scar.

Recovery from a cesarean feels different for everyone. It can feel painful because of the challenge that presents with caring for you and your new baby. Like any wound, it will continue to feel better and better each day. Staying on top of your medication that is provided will help reduce the pain of your cesarean birth incision and reduce healing time. Nutrition, hydration, rest, and scar massage with diaphragmatic breathing will support faster healing and recovery time with a cesarean.

Let's review:

- Birth by cesarean is a major abdominal surgery. Focus on rest, healing, and hydrating.

- Once your incision is healed, you can begin scar tissue desensitization to further support healing, reduce tissue adhesion, and numbness.
- Diaphragmatic breathing and deep core rehab are needed after a cesarean birth.

Postpartum depletion

Postnatal depletion affects more than 50 percent of women who have given birth. However, the majority of women who give birth are not aware of this depletion, what it is, or how to heal it. So what exactly is postnatal depletion?

Postnatal depletion happens when a mother gives all her nutrients to her growing baby during pregnancy and the breast-feeding phase. Postnatal depletion occurs as a result of growing a baby, yet there are factors that will prolong this depletion phase: poor nutrition, lack of sleep, and societal pressure.

The foods you eat during pregnancy and after effect your postpartum recovery. When your body doesn't have the minerals, vitamins, and nutrients that it needs, your body begins to suffer. This affects us mentally, emotionally, and physically. This is why focusing on a whole food diet and supplementing with a vitamin(s) is the most beneficial way to give our body what it needs.

Unfortunately, lack of sleep is part of the motherhood journey. We cannot always control this; thanks to our little human's constant needs. So this is a hard part to come by.

Society pressures can be very pressing and hurt our mental health as mothers. The pressure to do it all, be it all, and lose the baby weight is really pushed on new mothers in many areas. Many of us struggle with accessing time away from work. The workplace is very demanding and does not allow new mothers to honor their bodies or their babies as well as it should. This leads to burnout on the mother's end and typically brings about poor nutrition, more stress, and unhealthy habits in the postpartum phase, which continues to exacerbate the depletion.

Mothers who have more than one child have higher rates of depletion. Mothers who have children less than three years apart and mothers who have poor nutrition habits suffer the most from depletion. Some signs of depletion include:

- Fatigue
- Falling asleep
- Emotional exhaustion
- Mood swings
- Brain fog, aka baby brain
- Extreme hair loss
- Feeling guilt or shame

Some of these symptoms may be felt during pregnancy, even before the baby is born, especially if the mother is not well nourished before she becomes pregnant. There are women who will experience postnatal depletion for a decade if they are not aware of how to solve the issue. If postnatal depletion is not addressed, mothers experience physical, mental, and emotional symptoms that can lead to postnatal depression.

How to fix depletion. Lack of nutrients is the main cause of postnatal depletion. Eating enough whole foods with the proper balance of macronutrients, staying hydrated, and supplementing with vitamins is going to give your body the best chance at combating depletion right out of the gate. To recover and rebuild your strength, fuel has to be a top priority. Mothers are most deficient in B_{12}, iron, zinc, vitamins C, D, magnesium, and copper. Having a well-rounded diet in whole foods will provide an abundance of these vitamins in addition to a well-sourced supplement, your body will feel better and better over time.

Whether you want to believe it or not, our bodies and minds are interconnected. If our bodies aren't running well, our minds will not be either. Doing your best to take care of your body through nutrition, rest, and reducing stress will make all the difference. Be sure to get a support team together for yourself, people you can call on when you need it. This may be family, friends, neighbors, or a therapist. Ask for help when you need it and understand that it's okay to love your children so much, and it's okay to need a small break from them also. This does not mean you love them any less!

Let's review:

- Postnatal depletion affects more than 50 percent of women who have given birth.
- Having a well-rounded diet in whole foods will provide an abundance of these vitamins, in addition to a well-sourced supplement, your body will feel better and better over time.
- Doing your best to take care of your body through nutrition, rest, and reducing stress will make all the difference.

Diastasis recti

First and foremost, diastasis recti is a whole-body issue. It needs to be addressed as such, otherwise healing will become cumbersome. There is a lot of false information about diastasis recti, so let's first start with the basics.

What is diastasis recti?

Diastasis recti, or diastasis recti abdominis or abdominal separation, is the separation of the rectus muscles. The majority of cases present from women who have given birth to a child. However, you do not have to have had a baby to suffer from diastasis recti (see image 5). Research states that 66 percent of childbearing women will have an abdominal separation that does not heal after the initial eight-week post-partum period.

Research also states that 100 percent of all childbearing women will present with abdominal separation after child-birth. It is after the eight-week period that if the gap has not healed on its own or is causing pain, one must begin a specific healing process to retain a functional core unit.

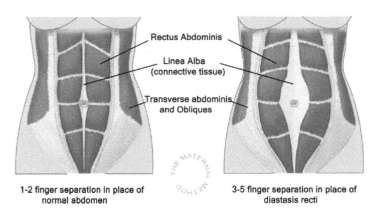

Rectus Abdominis

Linea Alba
(connective tissue)

Transverse abdominis
and Obliques

1-2 finger separation in place of
normal abdomen

3-5 finger separation in place of
diastasis recti

Diastasis prevention and healing in a nutshell comes down to how connected you are to your core unit and how strong the fascia is down the middle of your rectus. The strength of fascia is all dependent on how strong and connected you are to your core unit. This all begins with a knowledge of how to breathe, understanding how to control your intraabdominal pressure, and understanding what movements you do safely and which ones are not safe. It takes anywhere from six months to two years for your fascia to regenerate after having a baby, so patience and consistency are important in your healing journey.

How do you fix diastasis recti?

It is important to understand that just fixing the separation will not work. You must first adapt a few things in your everyday movements, such as your breathing and your posture. These are the crucial two steps one must begin to start repairing the abdominal separation. Not only will these two steps heal a separation, they support proper core mechanics in general. The hard part with society today is that social media sites, Pinterest, and Google are swarming with "healing moves" and "diastasis recti safe core moves." The issue with 95 percent of these is that it leads to the notion that by doing these particular moves, your diastasis recti will heal. The deeper level issue on this matter is that if you are not aware of *how* to do these moves, you could prolong healing or even make the separation worse.

You need to find, feel, and reconnect with your core unit and pelvic floor, and this is done by breathing correctly. Once you have connected to your breath, you can begin to engage the muscles in gentle rehabbing/restoration-type movements leading with your breath. Are you tired of me writing about how important your breathing is in helping your body heal?

Once your mind/body connection is there, and restoration is feeling strong, you want to work on restrengthening. Only then and *only* then should you move onto more intense exercise. It is best to avoid any sort of sit-up, crunch, or plank variation of movement during this strengthening time.

You want to focus on your posture. Stand, sit and walk in alignment, keeping a neutral pelvis to reduce intra-abdominal pressure, and don't tuck your butt or push out your chest! It is also really important to walk barefoot, without shoes for as often as possible. Our feet have become very weak. As a society, we are always wearing shoes; however, this affects your posture, which will have long-lasting effects on your diastasis.

Being aware of how you roll out of bed, get up off the couch, lift heavy objects (like your kids, groceries, or laundry baskets) will also affect your healing. Utilizing the belly pump to support equal intra-abdominal pressure is very important during these everyday movements. Through your healing, there is a general progression of movements:

- Supine
- Side lying
- Quadruped
- Kneeling/standing

Keeping this in mind, as you connect and keep your pressure equalized in supine, you can attempt to do so in side-lying positions, then kneeling, then side plank, etc.

Beyond the gap

Healing your diastasis is more about rebuilding the strength and integrity in your linea alba than it is about closing the gap. Many women never fully close their gap; however, they have a very functional core unit because they have taken the time to heal, connect to their breath, and understand how to control the pressure in their core.

How to check if I have a diastasis:

You can check your diastasis by yourself, you can ask your doctor to check you at your six-week appointment, or you can ask a pelvic floor physical therapist to check you. I suggest doing all three.

If you are checking it yourself, here are the simple steps:

1. Lie down on your back, raise up your knees, feet flat on floor.
2. As you go into a small crunch (lifting shoulder blades off the floor), use your one hand to feel with your index, middle, and ring fingers down the middle of your abdomen. Start from your belly button and go up.
3. Repeat but go from belly button down toward your pelvis.
4. Your muscles will close in. How many fingers width is the gap, if you are feeling one?
5. This will determine the spacing from each rectus abdominis.

You may feel the largest separation around your belly button, and that is common. If you have more than 2.5 to a 3-finger width, you have a diastasis that needs focused support. Having a 2/2.5 finger gap up to eight weeks postpartum is considered normal. It is what happens after this eight-week period that you may need to do more intense intervention. Always check with a therapist for best results.

Let's review:

*   Some separation is normal after having your baby. Our bodies are amazing and were made to stretch!
*   The integrity of the tissue is more important for healing versus closing the gap completely (this may never happen).
*   Ask for a referral to see a pelvic floor physical therapist for support if you continue to experience pain in your abdomen, pelvic area, or feel heaviness or

leaking. These things can be healed, and you do not have to suffer in silence.

Rehab, restore, and replenish

Postpartum rehab starts with your core. Every woman needs to do postpartum rehab whether you have a diastasis or not. As you have learned up to this point, your core is what keeps everything else firing at its best. Core rehab has a series of steps. It starts with your breathing. There are then a series of progressions that need to take place with the breathing in certain positions to gain back your strength. When you understand how to control your intra-abdominal pressure, no move is off-limits. What you will find is that you'll gravitate toward moves that continue to build your awareness in healing versus doing moves to just do them.

There are several other aspects of core healing not related to actual fitness or physical movement. That includes breathing, core regulation, neutral pelvis, digestion, and gut health which we will discuss in this chapter.

Breathing to support core healing

The first step to core rehab is reconnection with your breath. Why? Because your breath grounds you. It reduces stress. It activates neurons in the brain and allows you to feel into your being. After we have a baby, our core feels oddly misshapen, hollow, and empty. Our insides literally moved to accommodate space for baby. Breathing allows these parts to move back to where they belong. Breathing also brings with it a sense of relaxation, which is needed to reduce stress and promote healing of the pelvic floor. It is something that can easily be built back into your routine as you are feeding your baby or taking a moment to yourself. Breathing also brings more oxygen into your brain, muscles, and tissues, bringing about a deeper level of healing within the body. It is also the first step to healing your diastasis recti if you have one.

Core rehab is simply the process of healing and strengthening your core. Your midsection underwent drastic changes the last ten months as you grew your baby. Core rehab is simply physical therapy. Birthing a baby is trauma to our bodies. Yes, it is beyond amazing what we can accomplish, but rehabilitation for new mothers is not being prioritized in the world today. I do believe it is slowly becoming more recognized. But as far as doctor's telling you that you should do a rehab program is rare. You, and other mothers, are still deserving of this information and another reason why I have written this book for you.

Core rehab focuses on the entire core unit, which by now you know is your powerhouse of daily movement from your diaphragm to transverse, to back muscles, hip, pelvic floor, and even your glutes and inner thigh muscles.

Where the issues arise during postpartum is typically due to the pressure that is not equalized in your core. It could be coming out through your pelvic floor, which may cause the leaking of urine (peeing of the pants!), the low back pain, or it's going to come out through the midline of your core because those are the points that are now weak due to the stretching that took place throughout your pregnancy.

For those who need movement, keep in mind the best movement for your body and mind postbaby is walking in nature and core and pelvic floor rehab before beginning any type of fitness program. It is really hard with the Internet and social media today because other postpartum moms will claim that this twenty-minute-a-day workout healed their core and helped them lose the baby weight, blah, blah, blah, blah. These women are skipping over a very important piece of rehab. As mentioned before, jumping back into a program, if you will, will only cause pain, injury, and the like further down the road. It is easy to assume we can go right back to what we were doing before; however, keep in mind, your needs will be evolving and changing over the course of motherhood. What once felt good fitness wise might not feel as comfortable now. Be open to that, and be open to new forms of movement and ways to bring mindful moments to your day.

Let's review:

- The simple act of breathing supports the majority of our core healing.
- Slow and steady movement, such as walking, is perfect for movement after baby.
- What felt good before might not feel good after baby. Be open to making and adapting these changes.

Form/function

The entire reasoning behind postpartum rehab is that our body becomes out of alignment during pregnancy, especially if we didn't focus on training throughout pregnancy. To be honest, about 90 percent of our population, pregnant or not, do not function in a good body, resulting in an imbalance in their body. Over time, this causes aches, pains, tightness, sore joints, etc.

As postpartum moms, our bodies have become pulled, stretched, and lengthened in many different ways. Postpartum rehab brings our body parts back into alignment, resulting in feeling less aches and pains.

As new moms, we all know the awkward positions we get ourselves in, the holding of the baby, falling asleep with our head crooked the wrong way, the picking up of the car seat, and overall, the general bending and lifting we do daily. If you are not aware of it, your body won't feel good.

The reason that I bring my clients through a series of core basics, along with progressing into Pilates movement, is that it is gentle yet powerfully uplifting. Pilates focuses on core control and neutral pelvis in every single move. Because this is such a focus, we progress in a way that allows our body to regain its form and function in everyday life.

One piece of the puzzle, postpartum rehab brings proper form in your everyday life. Think about carrying your baby on your hip, bending over the bathtub, washing dishes, even sitting in your chair or on the couch, rolling out of your bed, sweeping, carrying groceries, all those things that fill your life outside of a ten-minute workout. The purpose of doing a workout during postpartum rehab is to be intentional about aligning and building your core four muscles, along with the outer extremities. So as you go about your daily life, these can continue to build. If you are not taking time to correct your form during your day, it's going to be hard to heal your body. The more you put it back into alignment, the better you will feel, the faster you will heal.

The postpartum rehab allows you to ensure your muscles fire and activate when they are supposed to, when your body needs them to fire.

Let's review:

- Core rehab supports your daily form and function, putting things back into place after baby.
- Core rehab ensures your muscles are firing correctly and when your body needs them to.
- Core rehab supports proper alignment and neutral pelvis, things you need to function and be ache-free during the day.

Slow twitch vs heavy weights

When moms first feel ready to tackle their body after baby, the world typically tells you to do some type of workout program, which involves lifting weights. The issue with this is that most mothers do not do their postpartum rehab. As they begin to lift, they do notice initial improvements but are not taking note of their form or function. Think of building a house. If you don't have a sturdy, strong foundation, the top part will eventually start to break or wear or crumble. Our bodies work exactly the same way.

As they continue on, they will hit a point where they are sore. Aches and pains arise, and they struggle keeping up because their body as a whole doesn't seem to be functioning the way it once did. When you overload your body with heavy weight lifting right out of the gate, you tax and stress already-stressed muscles. Lifting weights causes small tears in your muscles, and it requires proper rest and recovery. This is really hard to do when you have little ones to care for, which is why lower impact exercises, such as Pilates, barre, yoga, are much more suitable during the pregnancy and early postpartum phase.

This is where the slow twitch fibers come into play. Slowing your movement down, slowing each rep down, and eliminating heavy weights will enable this to take place. (This does not mean you can never lift heavy again!)

The slow twitch fibers are the base that you need to build before lifting heavier. Slow twitch movements support the building of your mind-muscle connection and the fascia. Fascia is the tissue that surrounds all of your muscles. It becomes very stretched during pregnancy, so proper care and recovery of your tissues and muscles are important to feeling your best postbaby.

Therefore, lifting heavy weights right out of the gate will not serve you in your postpartum journey. I recommend moms to first start with their body weight and then add 1–3 lbs. as they feel ready. Resistance bands and small loop bands are also effective. Bands are amazing because they make you work the muscle on the cocontraction and the contraction, both ways, which is what creates stability in slow twitch fibers.

Most moms like to have an exact timeline, like, "Okay, I'm three months postbaby. Can I lift 10 lbs. now?" Unfortunately, it does not work like that. Every single person will be different. It all varies based on age, fitness level before and during pregnancy, and how well you spent time in your postpartum rehab phase. By starting with your core rehab and working your way up, your body will tell you in time what will feel best.

Gaining muscle is a slow and steady process. So for my postpartum mommas, keep this in mind, especially those who are still nursing: You can have relaxin, the hormone that loosens your muscle fibers and joints in your body, up to six months *after* you are no longer breastfeeding. Not only is gaining muscle hard for a nonlactating woman, it is that much harder for a lactating woman who isn't sleeping well and is caring for a new baby.

In my research, experience, and personal journey, I have found that focusing on a combination of low-impact Pilates and barre exercises will provide your body with the best building blocks for your future endeavors. Both forms of fitness focus on that deep core, TVA engagement, stabilizing muscle groups, lengthening, and posture.

Pilates and barre are both practices that provide the least amount of stress on your body, which is highly favorable for any mother in the first two to three years or more of her child's life, including pregnancy.

Pilates is based on neuromuscular retraining for the core, which is why it is so important for pregnancy and postpartum. Joseph Pilates started Pilates in World War I to rehabilitate those who were wounded. The first Pilates reformer was designed on a hospital bed to support patients.

Barre is founded on principles of physical therapy and is excellent at engaging those inner stabilizing core muscles such as your pelvic floor, inner thighs, all three layers of your gluteus muscles, and hip muscles, which is why the combination of these two formats provides numerous benefits for those during the pregnancy and postpartum season.

Let's review:

- Gaining muscle is a slow and steady process.
- Focus on rehab and working slow twitch, stabilizing muscles,
- Barre & Pilates are great low-impact choices for early stages of postpartum to regain strength.

Postpartum nutrition and hormone support through nutrition

Hormone health:

Hormones during pregnancy *and* during the postpartum account for *many* of the changes in our bodies from breastfeeding to joint laxity, acne, gut health, mental health, muscle tone, and weight loss. Much of our postpartum period is being told all our feelings and anything weird that comes up, like acne, hair loss, or less sex drive, is related to hormones.

And I hate to break it to you, but so much of it is. *But* we don't have to settle for less than thrilling things and accept them.

After you birth a baby, your progesterone takes a nose-dive. Keep in mind, during pregnancy, progesterone is at an all-time high as it is helping your uterus to grow your baby and keeping your placenta going. Once you birth your placenta, all that progesterone is just gone, which is why so many of us have such a surge of unpredictable emotions. Progesterone will not start to balance and begin producing again until your first menstrual period postbaby.

Prolactin is another hormone that aids in breastmilk production. Due to these extreme lows and highs of hormone levels comes moodiness, anger, anxiety, irritability, and depression. None of it is your fault; it's just what our bodies are doing to adjust back to normal. This adjustment period is different for all of us. Eighty percent of women experience some form of postpartum mood disorders. It is important to note that this imbalance is caused by chemicals and hormones that are literally changing as a direct result of growing a baby. It's a lot to handle.

We cannot change these hormones from doing their thing; however, we can do our best to understand our body and provide it with what it needs to combat these changes so we can feel our best. One of those ways is through nutrition.

Nutrition during postpartum can feel so overwhelming. Unfortunately, new mothers very easily fall into the trap of wanting to diet and drop any extra weight so it appears they have not had a baby. So much of this is thrown at us via media and social media today. The majority of the world does not understand how to tailor nutrition to a postpartum mother; more harm than good comes from this. Typically, what happens is that mothers will attempt to reduce caloric intake, which has a direct negative correlation to how your hormones are fed and how you feel physically and mentally. In the next section, I want to share a bit about the diet culture and how harmful that has become to new mothers.

Let's review:

- Hormones account for many changes in our bodies during pregnancy and postpartum.
- It affects our weight gain, weight loss, and how our bodies function.
- Diets will harm our hormones and how our bodies function.

Postpartum nutrition and diets

Diet culture has completely ruined our ego. Society has put us in such a horrible place for body image and diet culture. We are conditioned to believe that weight gain is bad, that getting our body back after baby is born is a must, and the only way to do so is through a diet. Time and time again, I see moms with newborns on social media stating that they are going to give themselves a few weeks before they go all in with some program. Diet's during the postpartum period are not only detrimental to your health at that time of your life, but they leave us feeling really defeated and thinking our body is not good. But let me tell you something, *your body is good*, okay?

As a whole, so many women, even before they become pregnant, live in a constant state of negative thoughts around food. Correct me if I'm wrong, but I've spoken to hundreds of women and across the board—it is the same: thoughts around good and bad foods, foods that have too much fat, or this is too many carbs, or I shouldn't be eating this.

The first place to begin to heal this mentally is understanding *what* exactly the balance is your body needs while filling your plate with whole foods. We shouldn't restrict or deprive ourselves but in moderation. What if we started eating foods not because it's what the industry says but because of how it makes us *feel*? As a mother, I personally do not mention any food being bad or good to my children. They all know what whole foods are, and I like to share the benefits of different fruits and vegetables with them. For instance, red fruits and vegetables are good for your heart, blood, and building immunity. Every time we eat, it is always a topic of discussion about how the particular food is serving their bodies. This is the mindset shift I want you to start adopting.

Pregnancy and postpartum is a time when your body is working overtime. Fueling your body with the proper nutrients is crucial to feeling our best *and* crucial to honoring our body for its hard work. When you understand the process of fueling properly, you won't feel deprived. You will reach your goals, and you won't have to diet.

As already discussed previously, it is very important to focus on whole foods using the plate-it system that was discussed in the pregnancy portion of this book. We have to restore all those nutrients that were given to our baby during pregnancy, so eating enough of the right things so you can feel energized and focus on healing your depletion is the only diet you should be worried about.

A note about hydration: Staying hydrated is so, so important, especially if you are breastfeeding—more water means more milk! Be sure to always have a water bottle with you, and adding in some electrolytes or a squeeze of a fresh lemon, lime, or another fruit is a great way to flavor your water.

Let's review:

- Focus on whole foods and plate-it system.
- Hydrate. Drink water!
- Focus on fuel for my body, not deprivation or diets.

Weight loss while breastfeeding

I'm putting this in here because I know it is something the majority of us want after we have a baby. We feel selfish for thinking this, but weight gain is hard during pregnancy, and it is hard to navigate during the postpartum phase with all the other emotions we are dealing with. As mentioned before, we want to focus on that *plate-it* system, fueling our body so our baby can also be fed. The science behind weight loss is actually quite simple; it literally is calories in versus calories out. That's it. 80 to 90 percent of weight loss efforts come from nutrition alone, so don't think that you have to have the perfect workout program to lose the baby weight. You do not need to do keto, intermittent fasting, paleo, or become vegetarian. Those are dietary preferences, and you don't have to do anything you don't find enjoyable. The only way to successfully lose weight long-term is to understand how to put your body in a slight caloric deficit (refer to resources to learn more about this).

The nice thing about the plate-it system is that you don't have to eliminate anything out of your life. So if you're husband happens to be an Italian chef who makes the most amazing pizza, you can figure out a way to balance that all out and still eat the freshest pizza ever.

It is important to not try any reduction of calories until your milk is fully established, and you *feel* okay doing so. For many of us, a reduction in calories too soon after baby (even six months) can lead to irritability, tiredness, brain fog, and overall just feeling cranky. This is a clear sign that your body is not ready for this yet. I have referenced a few books in the resource section for you to look into when you feel the time is right as far as weight loss. The simplest way as a busy mother, in my opinion, is to be aware of your portion sizes, whole foods and prioritize protein (twenty to thirty grams each meal). It takes less brainpower to understand and achieve while taking care of tiny humans. Listed below are some whole food snack ideas.

Postpartum snack ideas:

- Nut mix (raisins, almonds, pistachios, walnuts, pecans)
- Apple with a cheese stick or some nut butter (think only two thumbs worth!)
- Sliced veggies with hummus
- Hard-boiled eggs
- Rice cakes topped with nut butter, or avocado and sliced turkey (nitrate-free)
- Deli turkey (nitrate-free) rolled up with a pickle or in a lettuce leaf
- Beef stick or beef jerky
- Smoothie with protein powder or collagen powder (*needed brand*), frozen fruit, and spinach/kale/cauliflower
- Yogurt smoothie bowl with drizzle of maple syrup, 1 tsp. dark chocolate chips
- Avocado toast with tomato
- Chia seed pudding
- Bowl of oatmeal with berries
- Banana oatmeal cookies
- Protein bites

Supplements

A note about supplements: We are overrun with the supplement market, which one is best, etc. They are important during pregnancy and postpartum because your body is taking care of you and the baby. Supplements fill in the gaps of a whole food diet and will provide you and your baby the micronutrients needed to feel your best. Supplements are individual to each person, so it is best to discuss with your doctor. Always look for supplements that are third-party reviewed. Please note the resource list in the back of this book I provided a few for you to take note of.

Weight-loss supplements or belly binders are not recommended at any point. These will do more harm than good on our bodies and are not sustainable long-term.

Let's review:

- After baby, remember, your body is good. It is just different, and this does not make it bad.
- Weight loss will be a direct effect of our nutrition, sleeping, and stress, so focus on feel-good movement for energy and the plate-it system.
- Supplements can be very helpful to support our postnatal depletion gaps and support our stress as a new mom.
- Our bodies need quality food nourishment to heal, provide for baby, and keep our hormones in check.

Mental health effects during the postpartum period

Mental health during postpartum is a real thing, and every individual has different needs, but it is a *need* nonetheless! No mother should be navigating her newly postpartum journey alone, nor should she feel she has to handle all the things. Becoming a mother is a huge transition, and no one can really prepare you for it. You just have to navigate it, juggle it, and find the journey that suits you and your family best. And as life has it, as your journey goes through peaks and valleys, so will your mental health.

I remember coming home with my first son, being so excited to be home, but at the same time, I was so scared to be alone. I remember those two extremes hitting me so hard that it made me sick to my stomach, and I cried. What was confusing about this was the instant feeling I had to cry or feeling like I couldn't handle something I knew was coming for nine months.

There are 8,238,293,892 things that go through a new mother's mind, from everything to baby care, to work life, to fitting back into your clothes, how to take a shower now that you have a baby, how to manage outings with a newborn. (I literally cried the first time I had to take my first son to the doctors alone, like buckets of tears, because I was afraid I would do something wrong or something would happen.) Most of these thoughts are caused by the excess hormones raging in our bodies. But several of us struggle with anxiety, and it is a very real thing, even if you never struggled with it before.

A few things that could support you as you navigate all of this:

- Talk to your partner, and tell him how you're feeling. It's okay!
- Grab a journal and start getting all this out of your head onto paper.
- Take a walk outside, with or without baby.
- Less screen time, stop scrolling social media. Studies continue to show how negative this is for new moms.
- Find a postpartum therapist. (Ask your doctor for a referral, something you can even start during pregnancy!)
- Focus on deep breathing, mediation, positive affirmations.

- Ask for help, and remember that no one can read your thoughts. Being assertive and asking for what you need is really important and helpful.

Lastly, nutrition and daily movement have a very large effect in supporting your mental health. Proper nutrition allows our bodies to feel good and fuel our babies.

Let's review:

- Regardless of your feelings during the postpartum phase, they are all valid.
- Ask for help/support.
- Give yourself grace. Early postpartum is a season. Things won't feel this overwhelming through all of motherhood. They do get easier!

Consistency

Consistency during your pregnancy and postpartum journey will provide you the most positive results over time. It's the small habits over time that provide you the biggest reward.

This consistency starts now! It is never too late to begin working on your functional body mechanics now that you understand the anatomy of your body during pregnancy and postpartum. You now have the knowledge and power to build better habits that will leave you feeling strong, healthy and energized.

Let it be as small as changing your breath patterns in your day, taking a ten minute walk on your lunch break, or doing some squats after you use the bathroom. I truly believe, the only way you can make lasting change in your life is to understand the *why* behind it. I am so honored to have shared this information with you. I hope it continues to change your life going forward in your pregnancy and post-partum journey.

Ten minutes of strengthening a day is a perfect place to start, which is why I have written some basic routines for you to get started with. Before we get to that, I want to share some statistics with you. Exercise during pregnancy can reduce your chances of operative intervention by 75 percent, and it can reduce the need for induction by 50 percent. With mothers who do daily movement, we are also seeing reduced fetal interventions and complications during childbirth.

Your health directly impacts your baby's health, and I hope the information in this book, as well as this mother-hood movement plan I have curated, will empower you to make small changes in your day that will keep you feeling strong and your baby healthy. Cheering for you, friend!

—XO Kaitlin

Part 4

⚜

The Motherhood Movement Plan

The motherhood movement plan (MMP)

I have created the motherhood movement plan to support you in your movement journey throughout pregnancy and postpartum. With a background in special education, I have a strength in helping others fit needed, realistic, activities into their busy day.

Adding exercise or movement to your day does not have to be hard or overwhelming.

The purpose of the motherhood movement plan is to support you in daily movement to support your body mechanics so you have energy, feel strong, and can reduce daily aches and pains.

Now I give a large range of reps so as to give you a number to work up too. If you are a beginner, I would start at the lower end and work your way up. Ideally, the goal is to *just start*. Don't let comparison hold you in the trap of not starting. Any movement is beneficial for you, and we all start with one single step.

Pregnancy movement plan

Morning:

- Five to twenty diaphragmatic breaths before you even get out of bed
- As you sit up, you can practice a nice belly pump. As you sit on the edge of your bed, you can do five to twenty belly pumps while lifting one leg, knee bent.
- At the toilet, once you're done using it, shut the lid (or not), and do five to twenty squats. Do a posture check as you go down into the squat. Brushing teeth is another great time to get those squats in.
- As you wait for your coffee or water to boil for your tea, you can do some push-ups off the counter, five to twenty reps.

Midday: Take a five- to fifteen-minute walk, or do some stair walking.

- Add in some more diaphragmatic breathing and belly pump practice before eating lunch and after.

Evening: Take another five- to fifteen-minute walk, or walk up and down your stairs.

- While in the shower, you can do some pelvic floor activations or releasing, depending on where you are in your journey.
- Before bed, as you're lying down, take five to twenty more diaphragmatic breaths as you say positive affirmations to yourself.

93

- You can repeat the squats, push-ups, and seated knee ups any time in your day! Another great one to practice is a standing wood chop to practice your rotations.

For beginners, focus on two to three days of strength training and one day of HIT and one day of labor training cardio. Starting with ten minutes a day is a great place to start and work yourself up to longer sessions as you can fit them in.

For intermediate levels, focus on two to four strength sessions and one to two cardio sessions, the same as for a beginner.

Labor training plan

These are some examples of movements that you can do for labor training movements. The idea is to get your heart rate up for thirty to forty-five seconds and then bring it down for a full minute or two before you perform another burst. During that down phase, you want to go back to your diaphragmatic breathing while practicing your affirmations and any other mental imagery that will serve you. These short bursts with rest periods can last anywhere between ten to twenty minutes. Only do what feels comfortable for you. Everyone has a different comfort level.

- Sumo squat taps
- Squat with bicep curl
- Squat to curl to shoulder press
- Kettlebell swing
- Lateral step touch
- Step-ups or knee raises
- Squat jacks (tap outs or small ROM)

- Lunge pulse
- Walking, fast walking, or jogging

Some days it may feel really hard to move. Try it for five minutes (even if you just walk up and down a set of stairs or around your car in the driveway), and chances are, you'll give a bit longer.

A few other reasons to stay active and keep moving during pregnancy:

- Fewer pregnancy discomforts
- Manage diastasis recti
- Relief from common prenatal discomforts, such as low back pain, sciatica, symphysis pubis dysfunction
- Less weight gain

During labor:

- Thirty-three percent less time spent in labor
- Thirty-five percent decrease in need for pain relief
- Fifty percent decrease in need for interventions or stimulations
- Fifty-five percent decrease for episiotomy
- Seventy-five percent decrease in need for operative intervention

Benefits for your baby:

- Increased health and IQ scores
- Improved nutrients via placenta
- Reduced fetal interventions during birth
- Reduction in premature birth
- Reduction in childhood disorders, such as diabetes, asthma, and other disorders

Postpartum movement plan

Even before your six-week checkup, you can begin with breathing and deep core activations.

- Diaphragmatic breathing fifty to one hundred times before you get out of bed or first thing
- Hydrate with at least 16 oz. of water.
  Gentle deep-core connection moves one to two weeks post birth, such as
- Pelvic tilts
- Bridge
- Dead bug
- Standing knee taps
- Small-range squats
- Wood chops

With these moves, you want to focus on your core connection to your TVA and activating that in each movement. These are moves that you do in your day, which is why starting with these gently will support your biomechanics.

Resources for your pregnancy and postpartum journey

The Maternal Method Blog: www.kaitlinspano.co
The Maternal Method YouTube Channel: https://www.youtube.com/@thematernalmethod
Needed Supplements: Use code MATERNALMETHOD for 20% off

Science behind weight loss books

J. Syatt and M. Vacanti, *Eat It!: The Most Sustainable Diet and Workout Ever Made: Burn Fat, Get Strong, and Enjoy Your Favourite Foods Guilt Free* (HarperCollins UK, 2022).

M. Matthews, *Thinner Leaner Stronger: The Simple Science of Building the Ultimate Female Body* (Oculus, 2018).

A. Calabrese, *Lose Weight like Crazy even if You Have a Crazy Life!* (Simon and Schuster, 2020).

Miscarriage and infant loss resources:

Share Pregnancy & Infant Loss: https://nationalshare.org/

Star Legacy Foundation: https://starlegacyfoundation.org/

- National Maternal Mental Health Hotline: 1-833-943-5746
  - o The Hotline, funded by the US Health Resources and Services Administration (HRSA) and powered by Postpartum Support International is available 24-7, 365 days a year in English or Spanish and other languages by request.
  - o Call or text the hotline anytime to connect: 833-943-5746

Pregnancy Loss Support Program: https://www.pregnancy-loss.org/

International Stillbirth Alliance: https://www.stillbirthalliance.org/

Miscarriage Hurts, Hope after Loss: https://www.miscarriage-hurts.com/en

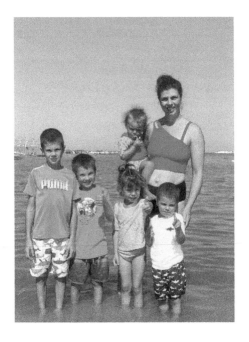

Who is Kaitlin?

Kaitlin is an author, blogger, wife, and homeschooling mother of five kiddos under the age of eight. She has the privilege of working with women throughout their pregnancy and postpartum journey. *She helps them prepare their bodies for pregnancy, birth, and a faster recovery postpartum so they can feel strong, confident, and have energy as a busy mom.*

After tragically losing her best friend to a childbirth related incident and struggling to find reliable information in her own pregnancy and postpartum journey, she began to explore science-based strategies that support mothers in the perinatal season.

The more she read and put into practice throughout her own pregnancies, she realized that moms needed access to these evidence-based practices. As a mother, you have the right to understand this information so you can prepare for a positive birth experience, recover faster, and stay strong for motherhood.

With this information, you will understand exactly how to navigate body mechanics to support your pregnancy body, help you prepare for labor and birth, and recover faster so you can have energy to support your family.

Kaitlin's certifications:

- BA early childhood education with a minor in human development
- MEd early childhood special education
- Holistic fertility and pregnancy safe coach
- Pregnancy and postpartum corrective exercise specialist
- Certified Pilates and barre instructor
- Pre- and postnatal Pilates certified
- Postnatal Pilates and diastasis recti certified

Acknowledgments

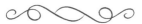

Christie, it was you, my dear friend, who inspired me to look beyond the surface for information that through the loss of your life, we can help many more.

To my children, may you always pursue your dreams and work diligently until you achieve them. Thank you for allowing me the time and space to grow into the mother you need me to be. (I'm still growing!) You each have such a special role in my life and how this book came about. It would not have been possible without the birth of each of you.

To my husband, who has loved me in all phases of each pregnancy, postpartum and new motherhood phase. You always believed in me and never once doubted my dreams of the mission in my heart to support pregnant and postpartum women.

To Catherine, Kylee, Alexis, Sarah B., Haley from Vermont Doula Company, my mom, and Marie, who knew I was writing a book, thank you for your unsolicited advice and encouragement through the process. To Sarena, my support person, all my book editors, the design team, and all those who unknowingly supported me in this journey, thank you. No words can describe how grateful I am for each of you.

To everyone who takes the time to read this book, I am so honored and humbled.

I read a quote at one point that stated that grief is the love that you can no longer give to someone who is no longer here on this earth, so it's better to channel that grief back into love and spread it out into the world. This book is a result of the grief that I have channeled back into love to honor the life of Christie to provide the knowledge, support, and empowerment that pregnant and postpartum moms so deserve.

References

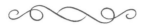

Acog.org. 2019. Approaches to Limit Intervention during Labor and Birth. https://www.acog.org/clinical/clinical-guidance/committee-opinion/articles/2019/02/approaches-to-limit-intervention-during-labor-and-birth.

Bowman, K. and Northrup, C. 2016. *Diastasis Recti: The Whole-Body Solution to Abdominal Weakness and Separation*: Propriometrics Press.

Cabana, M. D., Rand, C. S., Powe, N. R., Wu, A., W., Wilson, M. H., Abboud, P. A. C., and Rubin, H. R. 1999. "Why Don't Physicians Follow Clinical Practice Guidelines?" JAMA, 282(15), 1458. https://doi.org/10.1001/jama.282.15.1458.

Calabrese, A. 2020. *Lose Weight Like Crazy even if You Have a Crazy Life!*: Simon and Schuster.

Clapp, J. F. and Cram, C. 2012. *Exercising through Your Pregnancy*: Addicus Books.

Www.acog.org. "ACOG/SMFM Obstetric Care Consensus." https://www.ajog.org/pb/assets/raw/health%20advance/journals/ymob/ymob_consensus.pdf.

Dekker, R. March 20, 2018. "Positions during Labor and Their Effects on Pain Relief - Evidence Based Birth®." https://evidencebasedbirth.com/positions-during-labor-and-their-effects-on-pain-relief/.

Dugas, C. and Slane, V. H. 2021. "Miscarriage." PubMed; StatPearls Publishing. https://pubmed.ncbi.nlm.nih.gov/30422585/.

Gaskin, I. M. 2019. *Ina May's Guide to Childbirth*. Bantam Books.

Isacowitz, Rael and Clippinger, K. S. 2020. *Pilates Anatomy*: Human Kinetics.

Kimberly Ann Johnson. 2017. *The Fourth Trimester: A Postpartum Guide to Healing Your Body, Balancing Your Emotions, and Restoring Your Vitality*: Shambhala.

Matthews, M. 2018. *Thinner Leaner Stronger: The Simple Science of Building the Ultimate Female Body*: Oculus.

Osar, E. and Bussard, M. 2016. *Functional Anatomy of the Pilates Core*: North Atlantic Books.

Paolo, J. D., Montpetit-Huynh, S., & Vopni, K. (2019). *Pregnancy fitness*. Human Kinetics.

Syatt, J. and Vacanti, M. 2022. *Eat It! The Most Sustainable Diet and Workout Ever Made: Burn Fat, Get Strong, and Enjoy Your Favourite Foods Guilt Free*: HarperCollins UK.

Weerakkody, Y. "Inevitable Miscarriage | Radiology Reference Article | Radiopaedia.org." Radiopaedia. Retrieved May 1, 2023, https://radiopaedia.org/articles/inevitable-miscarriage?lang=us#:~:text=Inevitable%20miscarriage%20refers%20to%20the.

Www.acog.org. "Early Pregnancy Loss." https://www.acog.org/womens-health/faqs/early-pregnancy-loss.

Www.acog.org. "Stillbirth." https://www.acog.org/womens-health/faqs/stillbirth.

Www.winchesterhospital.org. "Threatened Miscarriage | Winchester Hospital." https://www.winchesterhospital.org/health-library/article?id=223394.

About the Author

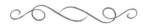

After tragically losing her best friend to a childbirth-related incident and struggling to find reliable information in her own pregnancy and postpartum journey, she began to explore science-based strategies that support mothers in the perinatal season. With a background in education and holding a master's in special education, she understands the value of evidence-based practices and realized that pregnant women were not receiving the evidence-based care that they deserved. When she was not tending to her littles, she became certified in pregnancy and postpartum corrective exercise, prenatal Pilates and barre, prenatal and postnatal nutrition, and several other certifications regarding pregnancy and postpartum care.

The more she read and put into practice throughout her own pregnancies, the more she realized that moms needed access to this information. As a mother, you have the right to understand the simple science of your changing body so you can put these practices into your everyday routines, prepare for a positive birth experience, recover faster, and stay strong for motherhood.

Kaitlin is the author and blogger behind the maternal method, a wife and homeschooling mother of five kiddos under the age of eight. She resides in Vermont on her family farm and can be found homeschooling her children, taking nature walks, reading, knitting, making endless meals for her family, and making trips overseas to visit her husband's family in Italy.

Printed in the USA
CPSIA information can be obtained
at www.ICGtesting.com
LVHW051630280524
781186LV00017B/388